Advance Praise for *How Not to Be My Patient . . .*

"This book is for everyone who decides to take charge of their own health and their own destiny. Dr. Creagan is a respected Mayo Clinic oncologist and now a brilliant author. He helps readers make the most important decisions of their lives. You will undoubtedly come to love him and his writing by the end of the book—but more likely, you will learn how to never become his patient."

—**Sanjay Gupta, M.D.**
staff neurosurgeon, Emory University Hospital
medical correspondent, CNN
medical journalist, *Time* magazine

"It is rare to encounter an individual who has the remarkable ability to communicate as effectively and compassionately as Dr. Creagan. Whether he is at a podium, visiting over coffee or informing you of your treatment options after a cancer diagnosis, Dr. Creagan makes you feel as if, at that moment, you are not only the most important, but perhaps the only person in this world."

—**Jari Johnston-Allen**
chief executive officer
Midwest Division, American Cancer Society, Inc.

"*How Not to Be My Patient* is a captivating, practical—and oh-so-compassionate—guide for those wishing to leverage the power of personal responsibility and to enhance their quality of life. Dr. Creagan blends personal experience, state-of-the-art knowledge and a passion for helping others learn to help themselves into a book that belongs on everyone's must-read list."

—**Michael H. Samuelson**
founder, The National Center for Health Promotion
collaborating partner, The National Dialogue on Cancer

"To have knowledge and a plan for using that knowledge in terms of your own health is very powerful. This book ties all the resources together."

—**Robert Dalton, M.D.**
oncologist
St. Mary's/Duluth Clinic, Duluth, Minnesota

"Ed Creagan is a skilled oncologist and a gifted communicator—working in the sometimes grim world of the sick—who brings a wise, witty, hopeful message about how to stay out of that world."

—Charles R. Meyer, M.D.
editor in chief, *Minnesota Medicine*

"Invest in your health by following these life lessons. Like *Cliff's Notes* for a healthier life, *How Not to Be My Patient* puts the current best thinking of the top medical professionals into one powerful self-help book. Comprehensive enough for a health-care professional but understandable by anyone, this book will add years to your life and life to your years."

—Marty Becker, D.V.M.
chief veterinary correspondent, *Good Morning America*
author, *The Healing Power of Pets*
coauthor, *Chicken Soup for the Pet Lover's Soul* and
Chicken Soup for the Cat & Dog Lover's Soul

How
NOT
to Be My
Patient

A Physician's Secrets
for Staying Healthy and
Surviving Any Diagnosis

EDWARD T. CREAGAN, M.D.

Mayo Clinic Cancer Specialist

with Sandra Wendel

Health Communications, Inc.
Deerfield Beach, Florida

www.hcibooks.com
www.HowNotToBeMyPatient.com

Library of Congress Cataloging-in-Publication Data

Creagan, Edward T.
    How not to be my patient : a physician's secrets for staying healthy and surviving any diagnosis / Edward T. Creagan with Sandra Wendel.
    p.   cm.
    Includes bibliographical references and index.
    ISBN 0-7573-0110-X (pbk.)
    1. Health.   2. Cancer—Prevention.   3. Diagnosis.   I. Wendel, Sandra.
II. Title.

RA776.C8126 2003
613—dc21

                                    2003050856

Publisher: Health Communications, Inc.
                3201 S.W. 15th Street
                Deerfield Beach, FL 33442-8190

Cover photo by David Sherman Photography, Minneapolis—www.DavidShermanPhoto.com
Cover design by Larissa Hise Henoch
Inside book design by Dawn Von Strolley Grove

TO MY PATIENTS AND THEIR FAMILIES
WHO HAVE SO HEROICALLY DEALT
WITH SUCH A DREADFUL DISEASE—CANCER.

CONTENTS

PART ONE: GOOD HEALTH BY CHOICE, NOT CHANCE— THE SKILLS YOU NEED AND WHY

PART TWO: WHAT YOUR DOCTOR NEVER TELLS YOU

PART THREE: ESSENTIAL STEPS TO SURVIVING
ANY DIAGNOSIS

LIST OF TABLES AND SIDEBARS

ACKNOWLEDGMENTS

John Donne was a remarkable poet who made the comment that "no man is an island." What he shared with us is that we need people, we need community, and we need support to go the distance. This is true in life. This is true in creating a book. Let me thank my community.

First I thank, and dedicate this book to, the thousands of patients and their families whom I have had the privilege of knowing over a thirty-year career. Each is a hero, each is a heroine, and each has pushed on in the face of numbing odds and incredible challenges that would wither the spirit of the most professional performer. I have marveled at how they have held their lives together in the face of a relentless disease called cancer.

To each of them I offer my admiration, my appreciation and my heartfelt thank-you. Let me also acknowledge their families, their spouses, their partners, their sons and daughters, and other relatives and friends who stood by them during depression, defeats and soaring victories. The 2:00 A.M. trips to the emergency room, the Christmases held in September as the clock was ticking. The son who comes home after driving forty-eight hours following release from prison to be at his mother's bedside. The daughter who rearranges her wedding so that Mom can be there. To each of them I say thank you.

My wife, my best friend and my partner, Peggy Menzel, has been with me on each step of the journey. Without her support, encouragement and critical eye, none of this would have been possible.

My three adult sons, Ed, Matt and Adam, are out on their own but were strong supports from day one.

Physicians owe their careers to many individuals who guided them. To my professors, my mentors, my colleagues, I can only say thank you for the privilege of your support and your encouragement as this journey has unfolded.

The first professional colleague to spend his time and energy in reviewing the initial manuscript was Dr. Leonard Gunderson, one of the foremost radiation oncologists in the world. Dr. Gunderson was the chair of our Department of Oncology here at Mayo Clinic and spent hours reviewing our manuscript. I thank him for his insight and counsel.

This effort also benefited immeasurably from the relentless review of Dr. Robert Dalton from the Duluth Clinic and St. Mary's Hospital. Bob labored into the early morning hours and provided wise guidance.

Peter Vegso of HCI Books pushed the envelope, went out on a limb and opened a door for us. For that we are especially grateful. We must acknowledge another door-opener, Dr. Marty Becker, one of our nation's most beloved veterinarians. It was Marty who encouraged us to push on, to put our words to paper, and for his help and encouragement a mere thank-you is not enough.

We have been blessed with a marvelous editorial team at HCI including former editorial director Christine Belleris, as well as Lisa Drucker, the editor who tirelessly reviewed every word, every semicolon, every comma, with devoted attention to the healing power of the written word in a book such as this.

Now let me turn to the one person who has been a catalyst, the flame, the engine driving this subject: Sandra Wendel. My coauthor is the consummate wordsmith, a magician with a keyboard and cursor. This all started as a casual telephone conversation several years ago. Without Sandra's tenacity, brilliant professionalism, and gift of pen and paper, none of this would have happened.

Edward T. Creagan, M.D.
Rochester, Minnesota

FOREWORD

Living Proof

[AUTHOR'S NOTE: *First, a word from one of my patients.*]

People ask me how I survived cancer. What do I do, they want to know, to stay cancer-free? My response is almost always the same. I live my life for each day and don't take much for granted. I treated my cancer like a common cold or the flu, not like it was a life-ending disease. With a positive attitude, some divine intervention, and lots of love and support from my family, I plan on living a long and healthy life.

In 1990, I had two weeks left in my senior year of high school when my mom noticed a peculiar-looking mole on my left shoulder. Our family physician removed it in a simple procedure. I thought nothing of it. Three days later my dad told me, "We've got an appointment with an oncologist. They got back the pathology reports on the mole you had removed."

Suddenly, it felt like someone had punched me in the stomach. I was supposed to be worried about things like what I was going to do for the summer and where the big graduation bash was going to be, not whether I had something seriously wrong with my health.

The cancer specialist told me I had malignant melanoma, one of the deadliest forms of skin cancer. The doctor seemed very optimistic because we'd caught the cancer early. Surgery was scheduled to be two weeks later, the week after graduation.

Nerves got to my mom, and she moved the operation up. The procedure was relatively quick, only taking an hour or so. All I really remember about it was waking up before the procedure was done and asking the nurse if we could order a pizza. Needless to say, the doctor was not amused or happy with his anesthesiologist.

With the surgery behind me, and the oncologist confirming that reoccurrence would be rare, my outlook was good.

So I successfully made it through my first year of college and went home for the summer. My plans included knee-boarding, boating and finding a summer job in my spare time. Halfway through the summer I noticed a pain under my left arm, but chalked it up to a pulled muscle, since I'd been quite vigorously lifting weights with some friends. About a month went by and things weren't getting any better, even after laying off the weights for the most part. Finally something clicked in my head, and off to the doctor I went.

With a quick physical examination, my oncologist knew immediately that a biopsy would be necessary to determine the nature of the lump. But at this point, he pushed the red button and said, "This kid's going to Mayo."

After all the tests and the surgery to remove the baseball-sized tumor in my armpit, it was now time to review the results with my new oncologist at Mayo Clinic.

Dr. Creagan walked through the door and introduced himself, then wanted to know what I liked to do, where I was going to school. He was more interested in my life than any doctor I'd ever met.

Instead of talking about the results from the surgery and what lay ahead for me, we talked about *me* and what made me tick. He had such a re-assuring sense of calmness and well-being about things that I almost forgot I was sick. He showed not only compassion but true concern for me in the true sense of a caregiver.

And then we talked about the news: He said I had a 95 percent chance of the cancer showing up again in less than a year, but exactly where and when, no one knew.

After leaving the clinic the first time, I had a million things going through my head. Is this the beginning of the end? My first odds were highly in my favor, and I lost. This time the odds were stacked against me, giving me almost no chance of beating them. Would I be back in a month, a year? Where would the cancer spread to next? Would I be able to live a productive life, or would this disease hinder me from enjoying the things in life that I loved so much (water sports, hockey, hunting, athletics)? Would I be able to have a family down the road?

After a day or two of really worrying about what could happen, I decided that was no way to go through life. I told myself that I would live my life as if I'd never had cancer and never would; despite the staggering odds, I told myself I would beat them. I wasn't going to let this ugly disease beat me. Besides, I still had to get back to school, and that was going to be far tougher than beating cancer.

Today, after eleven years of blood work, x-rays, CT scans and every other test known to man—and more than twenty-five trips to Mayo Clinic—I continue to be free of cancer. Although I now live quite some distance from Rochester, Minnesota, I still make the trip every six months to get my checkup and clean bill of health from Dr. Creagan. I could visit my local medical center, but it's worth the whole trip when Dr. Creagan walks through the door with a smile on his face and immediately reassures me that everything is okay, all tests are good.

Although I'm now cancer-free, I cannot drop my guard. Each time I step into the sun for an extended period of time, I protect my skin. Sunscreen is of the utmost importance. I don't apply anything less than SPF 30; most of the time it's SPF 45. The sun is a heck of lot more powerful than we think. Fact is, you can get sunburned through your clothing. I don't buy any of the special UV-resistant clothing, but I do try to wear hats when I'm out and almost always wear a shirt. Yeah, I'd like to go shirtless to beat the heat, but I'll take a nice farmer's tan over another bout of cancer any day of the week.

What really bothers me is when people don't seem to understand that any sun on your skin is damaging and that a suntan is *not* healthy—it destroys your skin cells and could possibly develop into a cancerous growth.

Another thing that I won't ever understand is people who know that something may be wrong or know they should get in to have a routine checkup, but don't. I see this all the time, even within my own family. It seems as if they think things will go away on their own, or they have the "that can't happen to me" attitude. Well, they are wrong. Cancer does happen, and it happened to me.

How hard is it to schedule an appointment and take a little time out of your busy schedule to get a simple exam and possibly tests? It could end up saving your life.

Each time I see Dr. Creagan I'm reminded of how special life is, and I thank my lucky stars that I'm here. He always lifts me up and helps me see the important things in life: family, friends and a conscious, healthy lifestyle. He has watched me graduate from college, fall in love and marry. Kerri and I have two sons. I only hope I can instill in my boys the mind-set and view of life that Dr. Creagan has instilled in me.

One thing always makes me laugh. Just before walking out of the exam room, he says, "Drive safely and don't forget to wear your seatbelt." He told me that the greatest risk to my health at this point is the drive to and from the clinic.

My visits with Dr. Creagan always seem to open my eyes a little wider and make me feel better about myself and thankful for all that I have going for me. I won't lie to you and tell you that I never worry about going in for a checkup and having him tell me they've found something, but very rarely do I dwell on the cancer that I had back in 1990. It may seem somewhat odd, but I am lucky to be his patient.

Chris Peterson

INTRODUCTION

He has cancer," they would whisper with pity and dread. The residents of my grandmother's rooming house would go to great lengths to avoid John G., the unemployed factory worker in room 212, as if somehow by just talking to him they would catch his horrible disease.

Most residents of 615 Hunterdon Street were down-and-outers, renting rooms by the day, week or month. Most were unemployed, but a few worked at a neighboring bar called the PON, Pride of Newark (a sure contradiction in terms), if they weren't on the other side of the bar battling with the bottle.

Having cancer in 1952 was as close to a death sentence as awaiting the electric chair from prison's death row—perhaps faster. What we didn't know then about cancer could fill volumes. But for me, a precocious second-grader living with my Irish immigrant grandmother who owned the twenty-two-room boarding house in the Ironbound section of Newark, New Jersey, being around someone with cancer was a defining moment—maybe not in medical history but in mine.

You see, the gentleman in room 212 had a colostomy—his bowels emptied into a bag on the outside of his body because colon cancer had destroyed part of his intestine. I was able to comfortably change his appliance (bag) and simply knew that I would care for people like this for the rest of my life. That was the way it was. No debate. No discussion. I just knew. This was my first experience with cancer. I was eight years old.

My first clinical encounter was as a second-year medical student at New York Medical College. The year was 1968. I was assigned an elderly black woman with advanced cancer of the stomach. Sunken eyes, hollow cheeks, skin stretched over bare bones—she was a living cadaver. When I first walked onto the ward and saw her, I thought she was dead. But I found the courage to approach her bedside.

Who was this woman? Did she have a family? What made her laugh or cry? What biological nightmare brought her to this dismal fate? I found it intriguing—fascinating in a morbid way—that one cell went haywire, robbed her of her future and eventually resulted in her death. She had no chance for a reprieve.

How did this happen? I was "hooked" on the journey to find answers to the cancer question. My classmates thought I was crazy to deliberately seek out the cancer patients. It was hopeless, they said. I was wasting my time and efforts. They were wrong.

A Disease of the Soul

I was initially attracted to the biology and the genetics of cancer and was intrigued with the notion of mixing various types of chemotherapy (chemicals used for treatment), then adding radiation and immune-related treatments. But it was soon obvious to me that my attraction was not a fascination with cancer as a disease of the body but cancer as a disease of the soul.

Over these past thirty-five years, I have pursued a path chosen years earlier in a grungy rooming house helping a sick and sad old man. Through him and the fifty-five thousand other cancer patients I've worked with at one of the world's foremost medical centers, I have discovered the majesty and the resiliency of the human spirit. I learn from my patients. I listen to their stories. And I learn to treat each day as a gift. A day not to be wasted.

In effect, the oncologist (the cancer specialist) becomes the spiritual leader—priest, minister, rabbi, for example—for patients and their families. I'd estimate that at least 70 percent of our time is spent simply listening to patients and hearing their stories rather than dripping toxic chemicals into their bodies.

As a physician, I'm inspired to hear the survival skills and tactics of patients who are at risk of being crushed by life's unfairness. It is their eleventh hour. And no governor is standing by on the hotline to commute their sentences. Those stories keep me going.

Every cancer patient is surrounded by a litany of emotional nightmares: the prodigal son who did not return; the wayward daughter who reluctantly comes back; the mortgage that is never paid off; the business reversals, shattered dreams and missed opportunities (especially the chance to say, "I'm sorry" or "Forgive me").

The most painful words I hear far too often are these: "I will never know how good I could have been. Maybe I could have made the big time, and now there is no time left." Yet, somehow, these patients continue to thrive and are a tremendous source of courage and admiration.

What I have learned from them is not to sweat the small stuff, but rather to savor each moment, to grasp it firmly, and to try to make the world a little bit better than it is right now. For me, each patient is a gift to be cherished.

Out of Suffering Comes Wisdom

The oncologist has "defining moments" every day if he or she takes the time to listen. Everybody has a drama. If we have patience, we doctors can come to know the human spirit.

We are each put on this planet to do something that no one else can do quite as well as we can. The lesson from thousands of patients is that everyone has a story. The overarching need of every human being is for recognition and acknowledgment. We want to be listened to, not preached at. We each say, in a special way, *Make me feel important. I am unique.*

Someone once said that everyone has at least one story good enough for a book, and perhaps this is mine. I write this book so that you can avoid cancer and other dread diseases. You have control over your destiny. You can and must take charge. As a patient, your job is to become the most empowered, the most knowledgeable person about your disease—because you are in charge of your decisions about treatment. No one has a greater stake in your health than you do.

"You're the doctor," some patients say to me, implying that I should advise them what to do. "No," I tell them. "You are the patient, you are in charge. Together, we will take this journey."

Sometimes, together, as doctor and patient, we may have to look at the relative futility of trying to treat advanced disease with current treatment plans. Many cancer treatments may worsen quality of life, and patients need to understand this reality. But let me be perfectly clear:

For some cancers, and other diseases, the track record with current treatment is positive, hopeful and holds the potential for cure.

Let me share an amazing story. It was 1983. I had the privilege of evaluating a fifty-six-year-old man for advanced lung cancer. He was referred to me from a prestigious medical institution in the Midwest. When I asked him what he was told about his illness there, he said, "They told me to pick out a good blue suit and six pallbearers."

He has returned to our clinic every year for the last nineteen years. He has the same blue suit. Five of the six pallbearers are dead, and his original oncologist is in a nursing home. He always asks me how I am doing. Astonishing! He has lived with cancer, and he asks me how I'm doing!

This is what keeps us cancer specialists coming back.

How *Not* to Be My Patient

I inherited my father's fascination with the Sport of Kings—thoroughbred racing—and eagerly await the arrival of the Triple Crown. Most of us know the names of some of these three races: the Kentucky Derby, the greatest two minutes in sports; the Preakness; and the Belmont, the 1.5-mile route in New York that often signals the end of many thoroughbreds' careers.

I learned a lot at the track—far more than from any courses in sociology. Rule #1: Be nice to everybody. The folks you meet on the way up the food chain, you will certainly meet on the way down—and they never forget. Rule #2: Never invest in anything that eats or needs to be repainted. Rule #3: Know everything you can about the sport if you are going to bet on it. Now what does this have to do with health and wellness?

The betting game comes with its own set of rules. The weekend gambler might just as well throw his money into the wind without some knowledge of the horses, the riders, the trainers and the tracks. The medical game is played the same way.

Consumers of health care need to understand how the game is played. Medicine is at the crossroads. There are presently 80 million baby boomers marching in lockstep cadence into their sixties and seventies, who will place crushing pressures on the health-care system during their older years.

As you well know, it's already hard sometimes to access medical care. Sure, if you have crushing chest pain and go to the emergency room in a major metropolitan area, most likely you will get excellent care. But if you have a routine, nagging concern, you may have great frustration just getting an appointment. You may not even see a doctor but a "mid-level provider" such as a nurse practitioner or physician assistant. Each plays a very important role in medicine. However, the sands of time are changing, and Marcus Welby, M.D., is quickly fading from the scene.

Another part of this drama is much less publicized. Bureaucratic strangleholds on medicine and a bewildering number of regulations are driving physicians to retire at younger ages and at higher rates than ever before. If you doubt me, ask your doctor, especially if he or she is older than fifty. Large numbers of patients need care. Fewer physicians are available to deliver care. And patients are bombarded with information on the Internet. What's a person to do?

Your Best Bet—The Daily Double

Here's the inside track. An ounce of prevention is still well worth a pound of treatment.

As we head into an environment of cost containment and the ratcheting down of access to medical services, you need every scrap of good medical information you can get to truly be in charge of your own health and longevity. Your best daily double against cancer and other serious diseases is still early detection of disease and lifestyle choices. But there's much more.

I'm going to share with you how to make the best choices, the most important medical decisions, you will ever make in your life. And I'm not talking about track tips or stock tips. By the time I see most of my patients, they have weeks, not months, left to live. Let there be no doubt: They are courageous, and we have many, many success stories that defy what we know about cancer. But truth be known, half of my patients never needed to walk into my exam room because their cancers were related to lifestyle choices they made along the way.

I'm not placing blame or guilt. There is little merit in looking back. I'm telling you the reality. The number-one fear of the person on the street is not heart disease, AIDS or arthritis. It is cancer. Public speaking is a close second, I am told. I can't tell you how to stand up in front of a crowd. But in this book, I will tell you what you can do, for yourself and your family, so you won't ever be my patient.

Although we cannot prevent all cancers and all scary diseases, we can place ourselves "on the rail" in a position to make the final sprint to the finish line. A guarantee? Of course not, but what I learned at my father's side at the track is that we can shift the odds in our favor if we have the knowledge to be proactive and involved in the most important race of our lives.

You can bet on it.

In these pages, I will relate many stories about some of the most incredible people I have ever met. I want you to meet them, too. But because of my deepest respect for their privacy and because of my obligation as a doctor to preserve the doctor–patient confidentiality bond, you will not be given, nor do you need, all the details about each of these remarkable patients. They are real. Their stories are real. And without them, I could not make this journey with you.

Part One

Good Health by Choice, Not Chance— The Skills You Need and Why

The Race Against Time

Time is the coin of your life. It is the only coin
you have, and only you can determine how it will be spent.

—Carl Sandburg

My father had a serious medical condition. He had an aversion to something called gainful employment. He was intrigued with numbers and horses and was convinced that there were reasonably predictable patterns governing why some horses won races and some did not.

He parlayed this passion into a career as a professional handicapper. He spoke in the argot of the shadowy world of the track. Terms such as speed ratings, track variants, post-position bias, blinkers, run-down bandages, maiden claimers and bug boys were factored into decisions of whether to bet or not to bet.

As a young boy, I spent many days at his side in pari-mutuel palaces with exotic names such as Pimlico, Hialeah, Saratoga and Gulfstream Park. I learned a lot of life's great lessons at the track. But one lesson that stuck with me in my later years as a physician has been the most valuable: Don't bet blindly.

Casual bettors at the track will consistently lose shirts, drawers and big bucks because they lack some understanding of the *Daily Racing Form*. This arcane publication contains reams of data on past performances of horses. My father did understand this. It's why he was a success. I never remember him working elsewhere, but I do remember him driving new Cadillacs and wearing six-hundred-dollar suits.

This may sound far removed from the exam room at Mayo Clinic where I see patients from all over the world, but it isn't.

Every day that you live, you risk your future by what you do. Or, in the case of most people, you risk your future by what you *don't* do. If you understand the odds, you can shift them in your favor. You cannot be a casual bettor. You must understand how the game is played.

None of us is guaranteed a future. You could drop dead tomorrow. Or you may live to 105—even if you smoke, drink, eat anything you want and rarely move from your Barcalounger. But, as my father would say, that's a long shot. Yes, long shots do pay off, but not as often as smart bets do.

How can you go where the smart money goes when it comes to your health? That's what this chapter is all about.

It's amazing to me that so many people bet on their futures unwisely by ignoring the health risks they engage in. Or they know the risks and hope for an unlikely payoff. Are you betting you'll be the one of one hundred or one thousand who lives long and healthfully so Willard Scott will put your name on a Smucker's jar for reaching one hundred—even though you avoid the behaviors that are known to enhance health?

Many of the people I see in the exam room lose this bet. Yes, genetics and inheritance need to be considered, but lifestyle choices play a huge role in whether you will develop major diseases. If a jockey or trainer gave you the inside scoop on a race, you'd plunk down your money without thinking. Let me help you make a wise bet on your health. Even my dad would say the surest bet remains an ounce of prevention.

Know your health risks and make smart choices. I'll help you stay on the rail and close fast at the finish.

It's your future you're gambling on. The smart money is on the right choices.

My Prescription for Survival

As Americans, we focus on high-tech toys to solve medical problems. The CT scan, the MRI and now the PET scan help detect disease at its earliest and most treatable stage and in doing so help people hold off the aging process. Could life everlasting be just down the road?

The spectacular popularity of medications such as Viagra to treat male impotence and Propecia to put hair back on our heads are evidence that we are increasingly focused on lifestyle medications to make us healthy and happy. Botox injections are wiping the ravages of age from our faces. If we just pump enough antioxidants into ourselves, we can surely fend off the free radicals racing around inside our bodies and making us old. Or can we?

Is this the secret to living longer and aging better?

Where did this attitude come from? Although the point is debatable, the eradication of polio through the Salk vaccine gave Americans the notion that big government, big industry and big universities would provide the panacea to put the genie of illness back in the bottle. Unfortunately, we as a society have really missed the boat.

We're demanding drugs for conditions that aren't even illnesses. Is pregnancy and childbirth a disease? How about jet lag or erectile dysfunction?

The *British Medical Journal* attempted to identify what it called "nondiseases." The aim was to prompt a debate on what is not a disease and draw attention to the increasing tendency to classify problems as diseases.

Several articles in the esteemed journal looked at unnecessary labeling of so-called diseases. The question is whether someone with one of these nondiseases may, in fact, be diverting resources (doctor's time and patient's money) from treating or preventing a more serious disease. Are these nondiseases in some way promoting hypochondria (imagined illnesses)?

The top twenty nondiseases as voted by participants in the *British Medical Journal* survey were these:

- Aging
- Work
- Boredom
- Bags under eyes
- Ignorance
- Baldness
- Freckles
- Big ears
- Gray or white hair
- Ugliness

- Childbirth
- Allergy to the twenty-first century
- Jet lag
- Unhappiness
- Cellulite
- Hangover
- Anxiety about sexual organ size
- Pregnancy
- Road rage
- Loneliness

We need to embrace the cold realities of life, of work life and of modern medicine so that we can devise a survival kit for ourselves and our families. Since when is aging or baldness considered an illness? We have plenty of diagnostic codes without adding road rage or loneliness. These could be symptoms of a society sick and tired of being sick and tired. These could be symptoms of a society fixated on smaller problems while missing the boat on big health issues.

Here's my prescription for survival: We each need to take personal responsibility for our own health and welfare to decrease our risks of developing disease, especially cancer. Let me explain. Most experts now acknowledge that at least *half* of all people die early because of illness caused by lifestyle choices, dietary factors and behavioral patterns. In other words, what you do and don't do with your body will kill you faster. You can lower your risk for premature death and disability right now—it's never too late.

And for those whose future includes an encounter with a life-threatening illness such as cancer or heart disease or diabetes, there is no doubt in my mind: **People who are physically fit, spiritually focused, psychologically intact and who have a support system do far better with their illnesses than those who are isolated and disenfranchised.**

The Best Medicine Is No Medicine at All

Mounting evidence from sociologists, psychologists and medical researchers suggests that strong social support—I like the term *connectedness*—can help you live longer. I know this to be true because I see the wonders of family and friends and pets every day with my patients.

A study of Harvard graduates from the classes of 1941 and 1944 identified the following common keys to a long, healthy life. These were men (yes, mostly men at Harvard then) who became some of the most prominent policy makers, educators, scientists and corporate leaders in our country. Those who remained productive through their seventies and eighties shared these characteristics:

- They had stable, long-term marriages.
- Through weight management and exercise, they maintained an ideal body weight.
- They observed moderate alcohol use, if they chose to drink.
- Regular exercise was part of their lives—and this was at a time before the benefits of exercise were really promoted.
- They developed adaptive coping skills such as a sense of humor and resilience, and were able to refocus their energies on art, music and other activities.

Social involvement is the most powerful predictor of living healthy as you age. We can also learn from the people living on the isolated island of Okinawa. The Okinawans live an average of fifteen years longer than we Americans do. Considering their lack of medical technology, they practically live forever.

For one thing, they are not obsessed with nondiseases. They eat a low-calorie diet. They engage in regular physical activity, drink moderate amounts of alcohol and, most important, they develop strong social networks and spiritual beliefs that foster a sense of well-being. Sounds too simple to be true.

This is not rocket science—this is human nature.

I hope you're seeing the pattern here. Work at something you enjoy, and you'll probably live long enough to cash in your 401(k), buy the lake home, see your grandchildren grow up, travel the seven seas or cross the country in an RV. Attitude matters. Pessimists die, on average, eight years younger than people who have a positive outlook on life.

We were designed to be joy- and fun-filled individuals. Do you enjoy eating dinner with a grouch or playing golf under the doom-and-gloom of a Chicken Little personality? If you cannot have fun or generate joy for yourself and others around you, you will have very little incentive to go the distance in the race of life.

Every one of us has things we like to do and are good at doing. Cultivate and nurture these interests to make life fulfilling and promising.

You can't just wake up one day, however, and see the world in a better light (or put this book down and miraculously have a new attitude just because I suggested it). But engaging in positive social activities will transform you. I guarantee it.

EIGHT COMMANDMENTS FOR LIVING LONG AND LIVING WELL

1. **Form stable long-term relationships.** Friends, families, colleagues, even pets, are clearly buffers against stress. Rarely does the isolated, marginalized person go the distance.
2. **Maintain ideal body weight.** Many of us struggle with obesity, and the health fallout is significant in terms of high blood pressure, diabetes, arthritis and stroke. Ideal body weight doesn't mean starving yourself to be something out of hard-body magazines, but it means eating sensibly considering your height, heredity and lifestyle.
3. **Eat a plant-based diet** with an emphasis on green leafy vegetables, four to six servings of fruit each day, fish and poultry rather than red meat (in moderation, if you must), and attention to unsaturated fats such as olive and canola oil. You don't have to be a brown rice and tofu vegetarian. Again, being sensible makes sense here.
4. **Engage in regular physical activity.** Let the experts debate about whether thirty minutes is best or sixty minutes is better. Just get active doing what you do every day and throw in a walk four or five times a week.
5. **Longevity does not allow for smoking.** Enough said.

(continued on following page)

6. **Use alcohol in moderation,** if at all. Although there is some evidence that a glass of red wine may be protective against certain types of heart disease, alcohol consumption can be harmful to many other conditions.
7. **Foster a sense of spirituality,** a sense of connectedness to nature or your higher power or some force or factor over and above yourself.
8. **Find meaning and purpose in life.** This is your reason to push on even in the face of adversity.

It's a balancing act: You won't live forever, but you can't live like there's no tomorrow because tomorrow is coming. You can prepare for tomorrow today by making smart lifestyle choices or changing poor health habits—it's never too late to do that.

When you make the right choices, you can take a licking and keep on ticking, even when life throws you a curve ball, literally. Let me tell you a story: My wife, Peggy, plays women's softball. She's years older than her teammates, but because she's a vigorous woman who is careful about what she eats and runs religiously, she's fit and healthy.

One hot summer night in 2002, a pop fly was hit to her in left field. She dogged the ball and was on it, but lost it in the lights. Instead of ducking for cover, she thought she had her glove at least close—until the elusive ball whacked her in the nose. She fell to the ground, seriously injured. Seven hours later, after extensive emergency reconstructive surgery, she was bruised and hurting, looking like a raccoon with her two black eyes, but alive and healing quickly. I attribute her recovery in part to skilled emergency crews, to equally skilled surgeons, and most of all to her healthy mind and body being able to take a punch and bounce back.

The same would be true for any life-threatening illness. The fitter you are, the better you will be able to withstand the curve ball that comes your way. And frankly, my own level of fitness stood me in great stead the night Peggy was injured because I was 250 miles away preparing to speak the next day at a wellness conference when the call came from the ER at 3:00 A.M. telling me Peggy was going into surgery. Jarred from sleep by the call nobody wants to get in the middle of any night, I was packed and out of the hotel in minutes, headed back to Rochester on dark two-lane roads for the longest drive of my life. But because I was healthy and in shape, I had the emotional and physical stamina needed to make sound decisions—and a long drive in the wee hours of the night—in the midst of crisis.

We never know what the future will bring, but we do know that the future belongs to the fit.

LIVE LONG ENOUGH TO CASH IN YOUR 401(K)

The big day has finally arrived. Your boss shakes your hand and wishes you well. Your colleagues gather around a cake and make small talk about landing the big fish in your retirement or joke about what you'll do now that you don't have to come to the office. A cardboard box is filled with the contents of your desk: your family pictures, desktop trinkets, snowball paperweight and stale candy. Your twenty-something replacement has all but moved in on your accounts.

One more stop: the benefits office.

In a few minutes, you will be asked to make one of the most significant and far-reaching financial decisions of your life: How do you want to receive your pension?

What does this have to do with your health?

Plenty. Because before you can make any decision about your pension distribution, you need to seek the guidance of skilled individuals such as an accountant, a certified financial planner, a tax adviser and—believe it or not—a doctor.

Let's suppose you are generally healthy with normal blood pressure, no diabetes or heart disease, and your mother lived to a ripe old age. For you, the annuity becomes a reasonable option. You could very well "outlive" the lump sum you are presented along with the gold watch—and laugh all the way to the bank.

On the other hand, you may have a serious medical condition, such as cancer, and let's suppose that your expected survival is limited to a year or two.

In that situation, a reasonable option would be door number two, the lump sum. You and your family would work with professionals to set investments in motion to take care of your family, despite the ups and downs of Wall Street.

(continued on following page)

Retirement decisions are not always as obvious as these examples. From a practical standpoint, however, I suggest you see your doctor around the time your retirement is planned. Some minor blood abnormalities or trivial symptoms might lead to a CT scan or EKG and a diagnosis of a life-threatening illness. In that case, your financial options would be clear. You may not be around long enough to collect your full pension, but you can make provisions for your family.

Life is complicated and not always fair. But before you sign on the dotted line, understand your health.

Essential Keys to Long Life in a Changing World

We are now in the midst of one of the greatest migrations in the history of the world. Approximately 80 million post–World War II baby boomers are not only moving over the psychological aging hill they climbed twenty years ago, they're on the downhill side, looking hard at the diseases of aging. At the same time, their "Greatest Generation" parents are happily living longer and not-so-happily experiencing the diseases of aging as well.

With careful planning, these years can be creative and nurturing. But if left to chance and without planning, these years may not be productive at all.

Let's look at our changing world and navigate our way to long life.

Key #1: You will live longer than your parents and their parents

- If you are a woman age fifty and without active heart disease or cancer, you can expect to live into your nineties. However, the last ten to twelve years may well be spent living alone because men typically die at a much earlier age.
- If you're a man and you make it to sixty-five, you can expect at least fifteen more years of life and, with proper planning, these can be productive and creative times.
- Midlife Americans at age fifty can expect to live another thirty years, according to an AARP report. That's almost nine years longer than your grandmother or great grandmother lived if she was born in 1900. Although today's boomers may smoke less, which is contributing to

longevity, they're more likely to be overweight. And obesity may take away any gains we've made in curbing smoking.

My message is this: Plan now, whatever your age, because you will probably live longer than your parents and their parents, and life is more fun when you're healthy enough to enjoy it. Disease is not inevitable. You're not "destined to die" of the same disease that prematurely took your mother. You're in control of your health destiny. And you can improve your health along the way.

Can you live forever? Probably not, even if you're frozen, but researchers at Duke University say the maximum human life span will reach one hundred in about six decades. Japanese women enjoy the longest expectation of life today—almost eighty-five years. But humans generally are living longer, and that limit keeps steadily increasing.

What we worry about varies by age and background. Americans think cancer is the most serious health problem facing the nation, according to a Harvard survey. HIV/AIDS and heart disease completed the top three. Older Americans (sixty-five and older) felt Alzheimer's disease and stroke were among their top-ten health problems, but younger Americans listed concerns about smoking and child abuse. For African Americans, deaths from guns, stress and diabetes contrasted with fears among white Americans about smoking, child abuse, drunk driving and drug abuse.

For the record, heart disease and stroke will kill more Americans than cancer and any of the other conditions combined. Half of all cancers can be attributed to lifestyle choices. This underscores the overarching importance of lifestyle issues and early detection to enhance our ability to cure cancers. A sedentary lifestyle, a high-fat diet, inappropriate exposure to the sun, and obviously tobacco and alcohol use account for about half of cancers and can lead to other serious illness.

My prescription for survival can help you live longer and better, but you must first address the issues that are holding you back. Prevention is, of course, my mantra, but I know that the behavior changes—even tiny ones—that lead to higher levels of health don't come easy. In the next five chapters [chapters 2 through 6], we'll examine whether you're ready to change, how to change, and what to change in the areas of exercise, nutrition, stress, habits such as smoking and alcohol use, and sleep. We'll also look at other lifestyle choices you make every day and find ways to get you moving toward wellness.

In chapter 7, I'll fill you in on the secret to living longer and healthier.

It's health screening. Some medical tests are worth paying for; some are not. But first you must give your doctor a checkup. Like a good marriage, the doctor–patient relationship is critical to success—your health. Together, what you know about your body and your health will change your health behavior for the better. It's a partnership worth cultivating.

Key #2: You have to be a smart patient because doctors don't always know best—you do

- When we need him most, Marcus Welby, M.D., may not be there for us. Like his colleagues, he retired early. He's on the first tee these days.
- *Mis*managed care has taken choice out of our medical-care equation. The search for Dr. Right usually takes us to a crowded waiting room with old magazines just to get our seven minutes with a doctor who has three patients backed up and four calls holding on the phone.
- Women are taking the lead in becoming empowered medical consumers. Women make three-fourths of the health-care decisions (for themselves and their families) and spend almost two of every three health-care dollars (that's about $500 billion annually), says the Society for Women's Health Research. More than 59 percent of doctor visits are made by women. They purchase 59 percent of prescription drugs, and 75 percent of nursing home residents over age seventy-five are women.
- The Internet attempts to fill the information gap but often falls hopelessly short of providing trusted, actionable health answers. In fact, patients can fall into a worldwide web of snake oil if they're not sure how to navigate the murky waters of virtual medical hucksterism.

When I was a young boy growing up in New Jersey, doctors not only seemed like old men, they *were* old men. Physicians would practice into their seventies. That would be almost unheard of now because of the threat of malpractice and the pace of technology. It is not at all uncommon to see physicians retiring in their fifties and heading off to the golf course or for careers far less stressful and more manageable.

One of the nation's largest physician recruitment firms has predicted that within sixty months (from June 2002), 80 percent of physicians will not be practicing full-time. Just as baby boomers need access to health-care delivery, the clinic doors are closing.

So where does this leave us? Welcome to the age of the empowered patient. You must learn to be your own best medical opinion because you are indeed calling the shots. In chapter 8, I will tell you things your doctor never tells you. I will take you inside the medical world and tell you what doctors know and what they don't know. There is no magic or conspiracy "not to tell" patients what they need to know. The system is tying our hands, cutting our time, piling up our paperwork and leaving us little time for the real nitty-gritty of medicine—and that's eyeball time with our patients.

You have to make us work for you. By being empowered, you can get the same medical information a doctor would give you; under ideal circumstances, you just need to know what it all means—for your good health and the health of your family.

You'll find out how to get the best from your doctor visits. Why spend precious minutes talking about how much calcium you need when you really want to discuss how tired you've been lately and whether those headaches mean anything? You'll learn why you need certain medical records with you at all times, which ones those are and how to get them. Your medical records can be life-saving if you know where they are, who's seeing them and how you can get copies of your information. Like puzzle pieces that all fit together to form a big picture, your complete medical records can be invaluable when you're trying to put all the pieces together. Knowing where your records are and how to get them is your job these days. Don't leave it up to your doctor.

Where to turn for that information is critical. Media hype and headlines can be misleading and downright wrong. In chapter 9, I discuss issues we were never taught in medical school. Medical breakthroughs and big-time cures are not taken lightly, and a study involving mice or even fourteen people in Finland may eventually lead to medical enlightenment for you, but it's not likely soon. So before you get your hopes up, put your guard up and learn to read between the lines when you hear about or read medical studies, especially on the Internet. I'll help you understand the medical headlines and teach you when to get excited and when to be skeptical.

Key #3: You can survive any diagnosis

The final section of this book tells you how to handle a serious diagnosis and even an acute emergency situation.

- You'll increase your odds of coming through if you know what to do first and how to take charge.
- If you can't take charge, you need to know how to call on a network of support for help.

I offer essential steps to making the best of any diagnosis—even if long-term survival is out of reach.

Whether they're trying to beat a difficult diagnosis or just searching for better medical care, patients frustrated with the medical "system" are increasingly seeking alternatives. Depending on the age group, up to half and more of us are currently using what would be termed complementary and alternative medical therapies: mind–body techniques such as meditation, alternative medical systems such as homeopathy and traditional Chinese medicine, biologically based substances such as herbs and vitamins, body-based methods including chiropractic, and energy therapies such as therapeutic touch and Reiki.

As in any endeavor, the alternative medicine world can be its own worst enemy, fraught with the proverbial snake-oil salespeople and smoke and mirrors—only these days Dr. Scott's Magic Elixir is cleverly disguised as a vitamin or dietary "supplement" with enticing names like coral calcium, blue-green algae and shark cartilage. You do have alternatives, and I will be among the first to discuss which work, which don't and which might, in chapter 11.

A Prescription That Works

We human beings are amazing creatures. With all forms of therapy—including the power of prayer—I've seen medical miracles among my patients. Things happen that go against everything I've ever learned in medical school.

Almost every day in the clinic, I see individuals who had dreadful prognoses based upon a pathology report, a CT scan or an operative report, yet they have continued to do amazingly well. A variety of sophisticated tests have been performed on these patients to find the key to their survival, and there does not seem to be a consistent theme from these studies. However, each of these patients does seem to have several traits in common.

I know this because I recently had the opportunity to review much of the world's literature on longevity and found three themes that seemed common to these long-term survivors:

1. **A sense of religion.** By this we mean individuals participating in the set of rules and regulations for certain belief systems, such as Catholicism, Judaism, Protestantism or any of the world's religions. Others adhere to a less formal belief system or have their own sense of a higher power.

2. **A sense of spirituality.** There are many definitions for this term, but the one that seems to work for many individuals is the questioning of the ultimate purpose of life: Why are we here? What is this all about? It is an attempt to find meaning, purpose and cohesion in a sea of chaos and confusion.

3. **A sense of connectedness.** These individuals typically have long-term meaningful adult relationships in terms of spouses or partners or are members of a community that gives them support and encouragement during times of crisis.

Thirty years ago, as a medical oncologist, I would see patients in their seventies, but that was most unusual. In the 1980s, I started to see patients in their eighties. Now it is not uncommon to see women—and men—in their nineties who are "dead fit," to use a racetrack term. They're candidates for aggressive surgery, radiation therapy and chemotherapy, whereas years earlier, we never would have considered them strong enough.

When I meet with these amazing patients, I always inquire, "Tell me, Mrs. Smith or Mr. Jones, what is the secret of your youthful vitality?" First they laugh, embarrassed, and then answer, "I don't know." At this point, I jokingly offer to reduce their bill by 10 percent if they tell me. Then the stories unfold.

They all have a sense of meaning and purpose in life. They feel connected to someone or something, whether it's a person or a pet parakeet depending on them for their own purpose in life. They feel a need to contribute to society in some small way. Maybe they help a widow friend fill out her income tax forms or drive someone to the doctor or give advice to a granddaughter dealing with tough times. Chapter 12 gives you the inside track on survival and longevity because aging does not happen by accident.

Enjoy what you do, and chances are you'll live long enough to cash in on your retirement plan.

My Thoughts . . .

Plan now, whatever your age, because you will probably live longer than your parents and their parents, and life is more fun when you're healthy enough to enjoy it. Disease is not inevitable. You're not "destined to die" of the same disease that prematurely took your mother because you are more in control of your health destiny. But what can you do to improve your health along the way? A lot. That's why you're reading this book.

2

Pack Your Own Parachute

If you wouldst live long, live well;
for folly and wickedness shorten life.

—Ben Franklin

The Biology of Living Longer and Better

Just as we in the medical community suspected, your greatest health-care expenses are driven by the lifestyle choices you make every day. My colleagues and I see the results of poor decision making every day in clinic.

When researchers looked at the combined medical costs for thousands of employees of several major companies, they were surprised to see that the highest costs were for these conditions, from highest cost on down:

- Stress
- Depression
- Diabetes, blood sugar levels too high
- Weight, too fat or too thin
- Smoking, current or former smokers
- Increased blood pressure
- Lack of exercise

These are easy targets. We can modify our behaviors and change our ways. But we don't. Why? Because changing behavior is hard work. If we're going to change the body, we must change the mind. As research has shown, the best results come one step—one tiny step—at a time. And it all starts in the mind.

I tell my patients to gently introduce small changes into their lives. These are called "points of choice." Make a small decision and follow that decision devotedly. Don't try to change everything at once. That way, you're much more likely to turn good intentions into everyday routine. You may choose to start with weight management and nutritional issues. For example, if you drink 2 percent milk, drop down to 1 percent, or even mix the two for a week or so until your palate gets used to the lower fat content. Eventually, weeks later, start dropping down to skim.

Or you may begin with short bouts of physical activity (note that I didn't use the "E" word—exercise). Spring is always a good time to start outdoor activities. If you live where you can plant a garden, with flowers or vegetables, the activity involved in schlepping dirt, raking, digging and watering every day counts as exercise. No need to run out and join a gym, pay for six months in advance, think up a great excuse every day not to go and feel guilty. Exercise can start and stay at home. It's free. I'll show you how.

If your issue is stress, perhaps you just need to take time to meditate, even ten minutes a day, and that could mean simply sitting down and reading a book that has nothing to do with work.

You have many of these "points of choice" every day: at home (in deciding what to make for a meal, choosing one cookie instead of two, even where to store toxic household chemicals), at the grocery store (what to put into your grocery cart, reading and comparing food labels), at work (taming your stressful schedule, working in time for a workout, making choices from a vending machine), in a restaurant (ordering a meal), in your car (wearing a safety belt is not negotiable). If you become aware of these points of choice, you can then start changing your habits for good.

Changing for Good

Action is the antidote to despair.

—Joan Baez

Psychologists say our behavior determines our health. But knowing what to do doesn't always mean you'll do it. It's the old "I know I should exercise but . . ." rationalization.

Change is a good thing, but only if you're ready. So how can you identify your readiness to change? James O. Prochaska, Ph.D., a behavioral-change guru, and his colleagues at the University of Rhode Island's Cancer Prevention Research Center identified these stages of change:

- Precontemplation
- Contemplation
- Preparation
- Action
- Maintenance
- Termination

"If you're not ready, it's like trying to make a garden without preparing the soil," Dr. Prochaska says.

Precontemplation

This is known as the how-you-gonna-get-'em-up-off-the-couch stage. If you're in the precontemplation stage, you're not even thinking about making a change in your life. What you might be thinking is this:

- I'll never be able to lose weight, even ten pounds, so why even bother? (Feeling hopeless.)
- I can't quit smoking. I've tried many times before and nothing works. (Again feeling hopeless.)
- Exercise is not a high priority for me; I don't have time right now anyway. I can quit smoking anytime, but not right now. (Denying there is a problem.)

To move forward from precontemplation is a huge step in the behavior change process. **Many people never move forward from this stage.**

Your wife nagging you to stop smoking probably won't work, and she knows it. But a major life event may suddenly launch your efforts to adopt healthier behaviors. The birth of a child or grandchild can jar your thinking. You really want to dance at your granddaughter's wedding or see your son graduate from high school.

I know a husband and wife who stopped smoking on the birth of their first grandchild, but they agreed that they would resume smoking when they were eighty. The thought that they would smoke again was enough to help them stop. They made the leap from precontemplation right into the action stage and never slipped back. So far, they've celebrated the granddaughter's high school graduation and anticipate her college graduation, and they are just a year shy of turning eighty. Of course, neither one is even considering smoking again. But it's the thought that counts.

The nurses who staff tobacco quitlines assist people who want to stop smoking. They know that many smokers who call aren't ready to quit yet, but somebody's spouse may have nagged enough to get the smoker to make the call. That's why the nurses use a forty-five-minute assessment questionnaire to screen in the serious quitters. By asking pointed questions about smoking habits, the nurses can tell who is moving toward quitting and the next step and who is stuck in precontemplation. In fact, those who are not really ready are not yet entered into the program but sent information and phoned in a month for another assessment of their readiness to change.

By using these stages of change, quitline nurses have an admirable 40 percent quit rate, which is far higher than most stop-smoking programs can claim. They know who will be successful simply by their attitude toward quitting.

Admittedly, we doctors haven't done the best job of helping our patients who are stuck in precontemplation. We simply don't have time to provide the kind of lifestyle advice they need to make a thoughtful decision. But even eighteen minutes of doctorly advice on exercise, for example, can make a world of difference.

Researchers at the Cooper Institute for Aerobics Research and at eleven medical clinics found out that a little friendly advice from the doctor coupled with health education in various forms, including behavioral counseling, phone calls, a monthly newsletter, a pedometer and a calendar, can make big differences in getting inactive adults out of the La-Z-Boy and into activity.

The study, sponsored by the National Heart, Lung, and Blood Institute and published in *The Journal of the American Medical Association,* involved 874 inactive men and women, ages thirty-five to seventy-five; a third were minorities. Although none had apparent heart disease, about 85 percent had risk factors such as being overweight or obese; high blood pressure or high cholesterol or both; diabetes; and 10 percent smoked.

Participants were randomly assigned to one of three groups—advice, assistance or counseling. Over two years, the advice group received an average of three contacts (just *eighteen total minutes* of interaction with a doctor and then a health educator) for both men and women. The assistance group received twenty-two contacts (or almost three hours of interaction) and additional behavioral counseling, a follow-up phone call, a monthly newsletter, a pedometer and a calendar. Women in the counseling group received forty-four contacts (for nine hours of interaction); men received thirty-eight contacts (five and a half hours), which included regular phone counseling from a health educator and weekly classes on behavioral skills to help adopt and maintain regular physical activity.

The surprising thing is that all the interventions—from advice to full counseling—resulted in similar gains in women's and men's physical activity. Researchers were stunned to find that a little help yields an important improvement (as measured in cardiovascular fitness testing before, during and after). At the start of the study, only 1 percent of the volunteers were moderately active thirty minutes on five or more days. After the study, 20 percent met the Surgeon General's guidelines for activity levels.

Sometimes a critical illness, surviving a heart attack or stroke, or receiving a scary diagnosis is unfortunately another way I see patients move from precontemplation into active behavior change—simply because they have to if they want to live. We all know friends who quit smoking after a scare with severe pneumonia leading to worry about lung cancer. Or the hard-driving executive who survives the heart attack and becomes a model of wellness.

It sure doesn't hurt if your doctor brings up the subject of your smoking or your weight or lack of physical activity. While some doctors may feel their patients don't want to hear more harping on the subject, research shows just the opposite. Patients are receptive to lifestyle counseling from their primary-care doctors, and they attribute behavior change to "the doctor said . . . ," according to a study conducted in Ohio asking patients how they felt about their doctor visits and about what the doctors said. Maybe that exam-room nudge is all you need. I'll talk more about the potential of the life-changing interaction of the doctor–patient relationship in chapter 7.

Knowledge is powerful medicine. It moves us from not even thinking about changing our behavior to actually trying on the behavior to see if it fits—and into the next stage of behavior change.

> *If you wait for the perfect moment when all is safe and assured, it may never arrive. Mountains will not be climbed, races won, or lasting happiness achieved.*
>
> —Maurice Chevalier

Contemplation

When you're in the contemplation stage, you're waiting for that magic moment—you say you want to change (stop smoking, lose weight, wear sunscreen, cut back on alcohol use), and you're thinking seriously about it. But you haven't taken the leap forward into actually doing it.

At this point, you struggle with yourself and weigh the pros and cons and hope the pros win. You recognize, for example, that if you get up from the dinner table and walk around the block, you can fit some exercise into your day. You visualize yourself going to a restaurant and ordering the lower-fat meal. You see yourself in your life as you practice the health behavior you wish to change.

How do you get to that magic moment? If we only knew. What motivates you? That's the critical piece of information in this puzzle. Is it wearing a size ten? Or fitting into the suit you wore when you were married? Saving the money you would have spent on cigarettes? Whatever it is, you must see yourself being successful. That will move you into the next stage of change.

> *Begin with that most terrifying of all things, a clean slate. Then look, every day, at the choices you are making, and when you ask yourself why you are making them, find this answer: for me, for me.*
>
> —Anna Quindlen

Preparation

Nearly there. You have decided to take action within the next thirty days. You're beyond thinking about it, you're ready to change. You're committed to change. At this point, you may even have an action plan. Smokers might set a quit date and begin reducing the number of cigarettes smoked each day. Future exercisers may tour a nearby gym, or check out a walking trail or buy sturdy walking shoes.

You've thought about the behavior change, you see yourself doing it, and now you're ready to take action.

Action

This is it. You are practicing the behavior change you thought about and prepared for. You're cutting back your portion sizes. Or you've stopped smoking. Maybe you check your blood sugar as often as your doctor suggested. You're participating in the warm-water therapy sessions to ease the pain of your fibromyalgia. Whatever action you have adopted, congratulations.

Success is its own reward. You may find yourself falling back into your old ways, but one Häagen-Dazs ice cream cone doesn't doom your weight-loss efforts. You'll cut calories on your next meal. Even a smoking relapse isn't complete failure. You learned from the quitting experience, and you may slip back one step before moving ahead again. Many people find themselves moving from the action stage back to preparation but not often back to contemplation.

Maintenance

Once you have incorporated the change into your life, you enter the maintenance stage. Everything isn't easy sailing, though. You continue to work at practicing your new behavior, but it's not a struggle anymore. You know what might set you back (a particularly delicious-looking dessert or a stressful life event), but you're wary of these triggers, and you know how to cope and keep up your vigilance. You've come a long way. Some people simply remain in this stage.

Termination

Temptation no longer rears its head. No way will you ever smoke again. Fried food, forget it. One drink and that's it. Buckle up without thinking about it. You're a regular in the Monday and Thursday aerobics class. This is the final step in true behavior change.

My Thoughts . . .

Change doesn't come easy. It's not always lasting. But it's definitely worth a try.

What are your targets? What do you want to change? Just reading this book may take you from precontemplation into higher stages of behavior change in one or more areas. In fact, because you're reading about health issues, that tells me you are certainly contemplating change somewhere in your life.

Let's look at each of the major lifestyle areas for behavior change in greater depth, and I'll give you my best thinking on what you can do to break down the barriers that are keeping you from adopting healthier habits and living a healthier life. You can start taking tiny steps and moving through the stages of change, because the best part about taking small steps is that they add up to giant steps over time.

When given the chance to live better and longer, do what my father did at the track: Put the smart money on choice, not chance.

3

Exercise: The Real Fountain of Youth

*Next to a leisurely walk, I enjoy a spin on my
tandem bicycle. It is splendid to feel the wind
blowing in my face and the springy motion
of my iron steed. The rapid rush through
the air gives me a delicious sense of strength
and buoyancy, and the exercise
makes my pulse dance and my heart sing.*

—Helen Keller
The Story of My Life

What Are You *Weighting* For?

I can't take out my pad and write a prescription for any medicine more powerful than exercise. Here's why.

When I speak to audiences around the country, I take a gallon of milk with me on stage. Why a gallon of milk? To make a point, because 70 percent of women and 25 percent of men in the audience will not be able to lift that full gallon of milk—weighing about ten pounds—by the time they reach age seventy.

After thirty, we truly are over the hill as far as our muscles are concerned. At that point, we start to lose 1 percent of muscle mass per year. So by age sixty-five, we have lost 35 percent of our muscle mass without weight training. Not the hard body, rippling muscle, sweat-in-a-gym type of weight training. If you have soup cans at home, you have the makings for a weight-training program.

Likewise, each of us loses 1 percent of our flexibility starting at age thirty. Balance isn't so great either as we age. The football running back assumes a crouched position for a very good reason: He is more stable and is better able to withstand getting knocked on his head. So, too, our older folks assume a crouch as they age—much of that is nature's way of creating stability.

The individual who does not have the flexibility to bend forward is at higher risk for falls, which may result in hip fractures and other serious problems. Take note: The most significant muscles you need to stay out of a nursing home are the thigh muscles. As these weaken, older people become unstable, they fall, they buy a one-way ticket to a nursing home, and their golden years quickly tarnish.

As a society, we have obviously become couch potatoes. Most of us don't get off the sofa to change the TV channel—we use the remote. An equal number of us don't even get out of our cars to open the garage door—we use the remote—and rarely do we walk instead of drive. Surprisingly, no one uses a remote to open the refrigerator door, but I suspect that's next.

We have become carnivorous and sedentary, and in some areas, at least 40 percent of people are obese. Sixty percent of Americans have no regular physical activity. This is especially tragic among children and adolescents. Interestingly, high school student Marty Liquori of New Jersey broke the four-minute mile in 1967. Yet it was another thirty-five years before a Virginia high school runner topped that mark.

As we've seen, long-term studies of Harvard graduates and longitudinal studies of aging in Baltimore unequivocally demonstrate that a sedentary lifestyle is as much a risk factor for early death as smoking, high cholesterol and high blood pressure.

Fitness and cancer

People who are inactive seem to have a higher risk for certain kinds of cancers, such as those arising from the colon and the prostate. In terms of colon cancer, for individuals who are physically fit, wastes pass through the colon faster. This means that less contact occurs between waste materials and the lining of the colon, and this may have something to do with the lower risk of cancer.

A high-fiber diet—once thought to be protective—may not shield us against colon cancer, but compelling, long-term population studies show that societies in which large bowel movements are common have reduced risk of colon cancer. Some African groups have diets with huge amounts of fiber. Rarely do they get colon cancer. We have no definite answers why, but we speculate that cancer-causing chemicals in the diet have less time to be in contact with the lining of the bowel.

Logically, then, a high-fiber diet combined with physical activity whisks the stool quickly through the colon. This is a delightful fact to bring up at your next dinner party.

Why a fit man has less risk for prostate cancer is not clear, but an ideal body weight may have something to do with the metabolism of male hormones.

So when it comes to cancer, there is no doubt in my mind that the physically fit fare far better with cancer than those who are unfit. Regular exercise appears to reset certain body systems, such as hormone production and fat stores, that are disrupted if you are overweight or obese.

Fitness versus fatness

Researchers at the Cooper Institute—founded by Dr. Kenneth Cooper, long recognized as the father of aerobics—made a distinction between fitness and fatness. In one study, men who were unfit and obese were, of course, at greatest risk for cancer, far more than fit men of normal weight. But if a man was fit (as measured by performance on a treadmill test), being overweight did not raise his cancer risk.

I'm not promoting fitness *and* fatness, but think fit and you will find the pounds melting away with an exercise program. The point is that exercise comes first no matter what shape you're in. Your shape will evolve as you shape up.

It's less about fat and more about muscle. With loss of muscle mass as we age, and without a reasonable program of weight lifting, our bodies are ill-prepared to withstand the assaults of rigorous therapy, should we ever need it.

People who have had a serious disease and were lucky enough to survive would have made better choices to stay disease-free, according to a Harris Interactive survey on health funded by the Robert Wood Johnson Foundation. Although it's good news that people survive life-threatening conditions such as heart attacks, it's tragic that it takes a major health event to get their attention.

But it's never too late to change your ways: Survivors in the survey said they are better now than they were before they became ill at getting regular preventive care (79 percent), eating a healthy diet (70 percent) and getting information about specific diseases (67 percent). More are getting regular exercise (42 percent), drinking or smoking less (39 percent), and controlling their weight (36 percent).

Why wait? You can start on your healthier path now.

A New Definition of Exercise

The real Fountain of Youth is indeed physical activity. But what is meant by physical activity anyway?

Stretching in the morning sun. Dancing to a favorite song. Strolling through the neighborhood park. Chasing a giggling child. These are the movements of a happy, healthy life. And these are the movements your body craves and needs, says health and wellness expert Peg Jordan in her book *The Fitness Instinct*.

Jordan offers a definition that is much better than mine:

> *Fitness isn't anything real or tangible. You can't go out and buy some "fitness." Nor can you store it, save it for a rainy day, or share it. Some people think that they will never have enough of it, although others would look at them and believe that fitness is the main thing they have going for them. Fitness is a concept, a word, an image in the mind, shaped by decades of advances in exercise science along with corporate-sponsored images and publicly broadcast messages. Fitness as a cultural phenomenon is controlled by a cartel that includes several industries, among them beauty, fashion, sports, sporting goods, and media. What is real is your life.*

For heart-healthy exercise, the American Heart Association advocates a gradual program so that you can comfortably walk and talk for 30 to

45 minutes four times a week. How much is that? Just 180 minutes of walking (and talking if you have a partner) per week. You probably use more cell-phone time than that each week. The benefits in terms of improved self-esteem, positive body image and a sense of wellness can be spectacular. You may want to run a marathon, but that type of torture is really not necessary.

The Institute of Medicine (IOM) recommends at least 60 minutes of moderately intense physical activity each day to prevent weight gain and achieve the full health benefits of activity. In contrast, the U.S. Surgeon General, together with the American College of Sports Medicine and National Institutes of Health, says health benefits can be obtained from three 10-minute walks a day (total = 30 minutes). So which is it: 60 minutes or 30?

No one knows for sure, and certainly an expert panel can't tell you what is best for you. The answer may be somewhere in between. Experts recommend that sedentary adults try to *build up to* 60 minutes of moderate intensity per day, which may also reduce the risk of weight gain over time and will provide additional health benefits beyond 30 minutes of activity per day.

Up to 50 million American adults are couch-bound right now. Anything to get them off the cushions and onto their feet is a start. Lasting behavior change comes slowly, so don't throw up your hands at the suggestion that 60 minutes is what you need and then do nothing because the barriers seem overwhelming. Start somewhere: Take the first step, then build up to your comfort zone.

Walking pays dramatic dividends in decreasing the risks of cardiovascular disease, stroke and probably the risks from certain types of cancers. Equally important, quality of life dramatically improves. Best of all, walking is free. Most people can do it.

And walking isn't the lowly cousin to running for people who can't or won't run. Walking, in its own right, is an excellent form of exercise. In fact, a study in *The New England Journal of Medicine* indicated that walking and any vigorous exercise substantially reduced heart disease in midlife women of all shapes and sizes, not just fit women. Prolonged sitting was the flip side of that coin and increased cardiovascular risk.

Work in a workout in everyday activities. Moderation is the key, but what really is moderate activity? Washing the car, gardening and even vacuuming are moderate activities that all count toward your daily requirement. But you can make activity count in almost any situation.

Take the stairs, for example. Posting inexpensive signs promoting the health and weight-control benefits of stair use in a shopping mall encouraged use of stairs instead of escalators. It seems so simple, so cheap. But it works. Stair use increased especially among younger and older people. And that's just one more way the Surgeon General hopes we will all increase physical activity throughout the day. The research on this was published in *Annals of Internal Medicine*. (I don't make this stuff up.)

Use It or Lose It

This is not a new mantra. I'm talking about lifting weights. But I'm not referring to the ripple-chested, bronze Hercules of the magazines, nor am I referring to a goddesslike creature with flowing blonde hair and a twenty-four-inch waist. I'm referring to you and me. This is one piece of the physical fitness puzzle that has been dramatically underemphasized.

Many people wince at the thought of lifting weights, but the studies are convincing and very user-friendly. A good first step is an examination by a medical caregiver to be sure you're physically fit. This seems rather odd because what reason could anyone possibly have for *not* exercising? But just be sure you don't have some type of heart disease or severe osteoporosis. In which case, I still want you to exercise, but you will need to modify your exercise—go slowly, and you should be fine. Second, if the green light is given, follow some very simple rules:

- Start using hand weights like barbells (soup cans are the frugal gourmet version of barbells and much less expensive) to determine the weight you can easily lift.
- A reasonable program is determined by how much you can lift with ease. Determine the maximum weight you can comfortably lift, let's say, with one arm. If that's ten pounds, you would take approximately 80 percent of that (or eight pounds) as the baseline weight for lifting. Or let's suppose a biceps curl can be done with twenty pounds. Eighty percent of that figure is sixteen pounds.
- A sensible program consists of eight to twelve repetitions so that the last rep is at the point of maximum muscle fatigue. You're really pushing yourself on that one. Most of the benefit of weight lifting occurs with only one set. To do multiple sets may increase strength but only

by a very small percentage. The biggest bang for the buck is with one set of eight to twelve repetitions.

- Lifting weights on an every-other-day basis strengthens muscles and can help avoid osteoporosis and other significant health problems. We are in the era of time crunch, so it would be far better to carefully perform one set so that the last repetition is to the point of maximum exertion, meaning you could not lift it even one more time.
- On the "other" days of the week, perform your cardio exercise—walking, water aerobics, jogging, cycling, treadmill, step aerobics—something that gets your heart rate up.

Lift weights, lose weight. Makes sense. Miriam E. Nelson, Ph.D., internationally known author and assistant professor at Tufts University's School of Nutrition Science and Policy, created news worldwide when her research results were published in *The Journal of the American Medical Association*. After a year of strength training twice a week, women's bodies were fifteen to twenty years more youthful.

With exercise and strength training and without drugs, women in her studies regained bone, thus reversing osteoporosis. They became stronger—in most cases even stronger than when they were younger. Their balance and flexibility improved. They were leaner and trimmer, while eating as much as ever. What's more, the women were so energized, they became 27 percent more active. No other program—whether diet, medication or aerobic exercise—has ever achieved comparable results.

Did I mention that these were older women? Grandmothers. Women who may have never exercised or had been active when they were younger but didn't have a regular program of activity as they aged.

Dr. Nelson's bestselling books, including *Strong Women Stay Young* and *Strong Women Stay Slim*, build on her research base and show how to get remarkable benefits from working out just twice a week. At the same time, you can boost metabolism and melt away fat. Because muscle is metabolically active and fat is not, when you increase your muscle mass, you're able to burn more calories, even when at rest.

If strength training works for women—and it does—men should take note. It will work for you, too. It's just that women have never thought about weight lifting as part of their exercise regimen—until now.

Step right up: Stretch your exercise program. You don't even need weights for weight training. You can expand your exercise sessions if you combine step aerobics with strength training using resistance bands. A recent study looked at exercisers who did twenty-five minutes of step aerobics followed by a resistance workout using stretch bands to simulate weight training. The result: Step-plus-resistance exercisers gained more strength in addition to boosting their aerobic capacity. Resistance bands looks like rubber bands on steroids. They're available in most sporting goods stores and on the Internet, and are quite reasonably priced.

This two-in-one approach gives a complete workout comparable to separate exercise sessions. The researchers, writing in the journal *Medicine & Science in Sports & Exercise,* say busy people can see real results with a three-day-a-week program like this.

And what about those ab machines? If you *ab*solutely, positively must work your abdominal muscles separately, you've probably been lured into buying an ab exerciser. If you've been up late at night watching infomercials for expensive equipment guaranteed to tighten up those flabby abdominal muscles, you may have already spent too much time—and money—on stuff that may not work.

The *ab*solute truth came out about the tubular metal devices with names such as Ab Roller and ABSculptor in the *Journal of Strength and Conditioning Research.* Researchers in California tested the machines and found they were no better than regular crunches (some of us know these as sit-ups).

Also consider the electronic belts that stimulate muscles with no pain, no gain and only a battery pack—that's another story driven by clever marketing. It comes as no shock that the Federal Trade Commission investigated what it calls false advertising for such devices as the AB Energizer, AbTronic and Fast Abs. This governmental regulatory group thinks a few million of these strap-on, do-nothing devices have been sold for up to $120 each. So instead of rock-hard abs, the only guarantee you get is that you lose your money.

You don't have to spend big bucks on a piece of exercise equipment to strengthen abs, and research from the exercise experts at the American Council on Exercise (ACE) confirms my belief. If you are going to invest in a piece of equipment, they say, make it a high-quality exercise ball, which costs about $30. These are like giant beach balls. You drape yourself over them, maintain stability and perform a wide-ranging abdominal crunch (sit-up), plus many other excellent exercises (make sure yours comes with an illustrated video or guide). Many other ab exercises, such as abdominal crunches, hovering (which is holding a push-up type position while resting on your elbows), and bicycling maneuvers, are *ab*solutely free—you just have to do them.

For best results, ACE recommends a five-minute abdominal exercise session daily. If one exercise is uncomfortable, try others until you come up with a variety that meets your needs. This will help train different areas of the stomach and prevent boredom.

No matter which type of ab exercise you select, make strengthening your abs part of your overall fitness regimen. You'll need them to prevent injuries, maintain good posture, control lower back pain and improve performance in other activities.

What I do

When it comes to exercise, you're more likely to do as I say than as I do, but keep in mind I'm years in the making. Generally I'm up and out of bed at 4:45 A.M. I head for the gym on Mondays, Wednesdays and Fridays for fifty minutes of either high-impact aerobics or a Stairmaster set on interval training at level ten (the highest workout). On some days, I will simply hit the road for an eight-mile run without the gym. Why? I just need to be alone.

Each of these exercise sessions is preceded by thirty seconds of gentle stretching and followed by one hundred seconds of vigorous stretching of my major muscle groups. On these three days I also lift free weights—one or two sets of about fourteen to sixteen repetitions with the final rep at maximum fatigue. On the other weekdays I run, saving the longer ten-mile runs for the weekend days.

Never do I lift weights for the same muscles on consecutive days. And Thursday is an easy "day of rest."

What do I give up for this exercise regimen? I need to be tucked into bed by 10:00 P.M. at the latest.

Putting Activity Back into Life

Society, of course, doesn't make exercise easy. "You find very few jobs today that require physical activity," observed Paul Ribisl, Ph.D., chair of the department of health and exercise science at Wake Forest University. "We've been so clever at taking physical activity *out* of our lives." Most

Americans sit down at work and move only their mouths and their fingers.

"We were given the gift of time and blew it," said Dr. Ribisl. "We've taken the drudgery out of housework and occupations, but we're too foolish to know the time that was saved should be spent on family, friends, self-enrichment and exercise. Our machine only works if you exercise it."

Yet we still complain about not having enough time. The Surgeon General is asking us to spend thirty minutes almost every day. Our bodies require it. Only 10 to 20 percent of Americans make time to exercise at recommended levels—a vital component in weight loss and maintenance.

One step at a time is good walking.
—Chinese Proverb

It's never too late to exercise. Researchers always suspected that brisk walking would outrun, or at least be comparable to, other exercise, and an eight-year study published in *The New England Journal of Medicine* of thousands of female nurses is strong evidence. Women in the study who became active in middle adulthood *or later* were able to lower their risk for coronary heart disease just by brisk walking three or more hours per week (at a pace of at least three miles per hour or a mile in twenty minutes).

So take thirty minutes each day. You'll get the same heart-healthy benefits as those who exercise vigorously, and walking is easy and free. You just need a pair of comfortable shoes.

TOP TWENTY-FIVE REASONS TO EXERCISE

1. Strengthens heart muscle.
2. Decreases the incidence of heart attack.
3. Reduces risks for heart disease, including reduced LDL (bad) cholesterol and increased HDL (good) cholesterol.
4. Improves circulation and oxygen/nutrient transport throughout the body.
5. Helps lose weight and keep it off.
6. Improves breathing efficiency.
7. Strengthens and tones muscles and improves appearance.
8. Helps prevent back problems and back pain.
9. Improves posture.
10. Strengthens bones and helps reduce risk of osteoporosis.
11. Strengthens the tissues around the joints and reduces joint discomfort and arthritis if appropriate exercise is selected and properly performed.
12. Decreases risk for several types of cancer.
13. Improves immune function, which decreases risk for infectious diseases.
14. Maintains physical and mental functions throughout the second half of life.
15. Increases self-confidence and self-esteem.
16. Boosts energy and increases productivity.
17. Improves sleep.
18. Helps create a positive attitude about life.
19. Reduces anxiety and depression.
20. Increases resistance to fatigue.
21. May lengthen life span.
22. Reduces blood pressure.
23. Decreases the incidence of type 2 diabetes.
24. Reduces stress.
25. Improves cognitive function (you can think more clearly).

How many more reasons do you need?

Reprinted with permission from *Physical Fitness: Guidelines for Success* (revised ©2002) by JoAnn Eickhoff-Shemek, Ph.D., and Kris Berg, Ed.D., University of Nebraska-Omaha.

Daily tasks are not a chore, unless you can't do them. Opening a jar of pickles, getting up out of a chair, climbing a flight of stairs . . . they seem like simple daily activities—but if you don't have the muscle strength to do them, you can lose your independence, and your quality of life may never be the same.

A study reported in *Medicine & Science in Sports & Exercise* found that healthy adults who actively maintain their strength throughout their lives will prevent or minimize loss of ability to do daily household activities. Muscles begin to lose their strength in middle-age, according to researchers from the Cooper Institute for Aerobics Research. But muscle loss from inactivity can actually be reversed by exercise and strength training, no matter what your age.

Exercise, at every level, works. Until new research was done, no one had figured out how much older men and women should exercise and what types of activities are best. If you are in your sixties and seventies and in good health, researchers now say vigorous aerobic exercise may help your cardiovascular health.

Generally, it is recommended that older adults burn about two hundred calories each day through exercise. A study, published in the *Journal of Clinical Endocrinology and Metabolism,* found that participants with the greatest aerobic capacity (the body's ability to transport and use oxygen) were leaner and had lower cholesterol and insulin levels than others. Short bursts of exercise that get the heart and lungs working at peak capacity may benefit elderly hearts more than frequent, moderate activity.

Moderate activity, however, burns calories, too. And low-intensity exercise helps regulate weight and protects against type 2 diabetes. Do what feels right for you, but get your doctor's approval before you make a drastic change in your type of exercise.

WHICH EXERCISE IS RIGHT FOR YOU?

ACTIVITY	PROS	CONS
Walking	Can be done almost anywhere. Excellent beginner activity. Minimal stress to joints. Develops and maintains aerobic fitness for most adults.	For the highly fit, may not be intense enough to reach target heart rate range.
Jogging/Running	Requires no special equipment except proper shoes. Can be done almost anywhere.	May stress joints. Safety issues when done on streets and uneven surfaces.
Swimming	Excellent overall conditioner. Minimal stress to most joints.	Need access to a pool.
Bicycling/Stationary Cycling	Exercises large muscles in legs. Minimal stress to most joints. Can be done indoors.	Outdoor: safety issues. Indoor: need access to equipment; can be boring
Aerobic Dance/ Step Aerobics	Excellent overall conditioner if properly designed. Music and group exercise make it enjoyable.	Requires instruction. High impact can stress joints.
Rowing	Exercise upper and lower body muscles. Minimal stress on joints if done properly. Effective for aerobic and muscle fitness.	Need access to equipment.
Stair Climber	Exercises large muscles in legs. Minimal stress on joints.	Need access to equipment.
Rope Jumping	Can be done almost anywhere. Inexpensive.	Difficult to sustain unless fairly fit. Stresses joints. Skill required for effectiveness.

Reprinted with permission from *Physical Fitness: Guidelines for Success* (revised ©2002) by JoAnn M. Eickhoff-Shemek, Ph.D., and Kris E. Berg, Ed.D., University of Nebraska-Omaha.

Run with Your Exercise, Don't Let It Run You

Walking is easy. No special equipment is required. But fitness centers, if you choose to exercise there, can be downright overwhelming. If you're new to this, you'll want to get help because, frankly, you'll need it.

Some new exercisers turn to personal trainers, and I think that's a great idea. You don't have to commit to a personal trainer week after week, but tap into their expertise to assess your level of fitness and to set up a personal exercise prescription and goals. Meet with a trainer for a few sessions and let the trainer show you how to safely use all the exercise equipment and monitor you for a time or two, until you feel comfortable loading up the hip sled with fifty-pounders and setting out on your own on the gym floor.

But be careful. Anybody can hang out a shingle and claim to be a personal trainer. It's the certification that should make all the difference—to you. So before you sign on with a personal trainer, ask two key questions and make sure you're satisfied that the person who's going to make you sweat is qualified to do so:

1. Do you have a college degree in exercise science?
2. Are you certified by the American College of Sports Medicine (ACSM) or the National Strength and Conditioning Association (NSCA)?

Researchers in the *Journal of Strength and Conditioning Research* measured the relationship between education, experience and actual knowledge of nutrition, health screening, fitness testing, exercise prescription and general training expertise for special populations.

They found that a bachelor's degree in exercise science and certification with ACSM or NSCA, organizations whose credentialing is widely accepted, were strong predictors of the personal trainer's knowledge. Number of years of training experience didn't necessarily mean a trainer was more knowledgeable. In other words, this education and credentialing better prepares personal trainers to develop an optimal fitness program for you and will help you avoid unnecessary injuries during your workouts.

If your trainer or the fitness center staff start talking to you about nutritional or dietary supplements, steer clear. You don't need them, and you certainly don't need that kind of advice from people who are not qualified to discuss nutrition.

Actually, I'm not trained in nutrition either. They don't teach future doctors about that in medical school. I'm happy to say that everything I know about nutrition I learned from my wife, Peggy. She happens to be a registered dietitian with Mayo Clinic and works with people who are recovering from heart attacks. By surviving their heart attacks (and a third of people who have one don't survive), these lucky souls are particularly motivated to start eating well. Chances are what they have eaten or not eaten has brought them into our clinic in the first place. Peggy tries to help them help themselves. That's why I worked closely with her developing the next chapter: nutrition.

My Thoughts . . .

I am a marathoner. Growing up as a skinny little kid in New Jersey, I was told that since I had no dates, no social skills and no athletic talents, I better become a distance runner. I am fortunate to be orthopedically gifted and have run multiple marathons and have been able to run almost every day for over fifty years.

In training for a marathon, it is not a question of wishful thinking. I map out a plan and work out day by day, week by week, month by month, so that when the gun goes off on the starting line and I am looking down the barrel of 26.2 miles, I am physically prepared to go the distance—and mentally ready. I have to visualize my goal and take those small successes one step at a time.

It is impossible to envision running 26.2 miles. But if I see myself running the first 5 miles, the second 5 miles, and so on, I can do it. At mile 20, many of my colleagues hit the wall—a runner's term for thinking you just can't take one more step. But we runners **do** take that painful step. We press on even though we think we can't. And you can, too. For me, that 20-mile marker means I have only 6.2 miles to go. That is 10,000 meters or 10K, which is a common distance run for road races. I can grind it out because I have done my homework, and I am prepared.

The lesson is that we all must run small races. In doing so, see yourself winning and moving on. You can make your "pulse dance and your heart sing." Then you'll never hit the wall.

4

Nutrition: You Are What You Put in Your Grocery Cart

We are indeed much more than what we eat,
but what we eat can nevertheless help us
to be much more than what we are.

—Adelle Davis

Ladies Home Journal sent a reporter and a photographer to follow my wife, Peggy, and me around the grocery store. The story they eventually printed in the March 2002 issue was rather short. So let me give you the long version—with lots of important information before we get to the store—because, as Peggy reminds me every day, we really are what we put in our grocery carts.

Peggy is a registered dietitian. Those who come in with serious heart problems, once they leave the cardiac-care units, meet with Peggy to discuss the eating habits that may have led to their heart disease. If they didn't know before, they leave our Rochester campus armed with the best information available on food content and dietary choices, and a renewed sense of empowerment that they can make positive changes in their diets.

Like all behavior, you need a good reason to change your eating habits. Being a patient in a cardiac unit is one. Being overweight is another of those reasons. As the second leading cause of death, obesity, like the number-one cause (smoking), can be prevented.

There's a distinction between being "overweight" and being "obese." In adults, obesity can be defined as a waist circumference greater than forty inches for men and thirty-five inches for women. You don't actually need a tape measure to figure this one out.

A fourth of the population is currently on a "diet," and another 47 percent are making conscious efforts to control their weight, according to a national survey released by the Calorie Control Council, a nonprofit association of manufacturers of low-calorie, reduced-fat, and light foods and beverages. This is an interesting group to be talking about diets. Theoretically, so-called "light" foods should have contributed to a shrinking of America instead of its widening. But "reduced-fat," "fewer calories" and "light" gave eaters a false promise of easy weight control. Low-fat cookies still contain calories, and therein lies the problem.

I'm not laying blame for an epidemic of obesity in America, but a few years ago when Yankee Stadium yanked out its seats and replaced them with fewer yet wider seats to accommodate its growing fans, we better take that as a wake-up call.

Perhaps it's time we concentrate less on "diet" and "dieting" and more on permanent behavior change habits regarding healthy eating. Successful weight management will follow.

We've all seen (and maybe tried) the popular quick-fix diets. All diets work, by the way. But what is their logical conclusion? That you starve yourself, feel deprived and continue to drop weight, until you weigh nothing? Maintaining an ideal body weight (ideal for you, not for a fashion model or movie star) means a lifelong commitment to healthful eating, not an on-again, off-again scheme.

At Mayo Clinic, we are often asked about the Mayo Clinic Diet. It's an Internet hoax, an urban legend. These "miracle" diets have been circulating erroneously and have nothing to do with our clinic, by the way. When asked about them, we say, "There's no such thing." What we offer is a sound eating plan for life.

Calories Really Do Count

A hundred years of research and thousands of studies later, the role of eating habits remains the leading predictor of weight. But how we're getting those calories and what our bodies are doing with them seems to be a moving target.

In our new battle against the bulge, we need to muster the same health campaigns that have helped inform and nudge Americans to stop smoking, control high blood pressure and know their cholesterol numbers. Being overweight or obese negatively influences other disorders such as diabetes and cancer. Reverse one, and the others will be less troublesome.

We live in a world of fast food and fat food. Americans have become complacent about the fat in foods, according to some trend analysts. Through clever marketing, we're less concerned about the fat content in our foods, the surveys say.

Capitalizing on that trend, many brand names have literally rolled out highly popular and highly packed calorie- and fat-dense cheesecake snack bars and microwaveable calzone sandwiches. This is how food manufacturers sometimes make it difficult for us to make healthy choices.

Calories *do* count for most people, and what is crucial is caloric density, which is the number of calories packed into a measured volume of food. A tiny little Halloween-sized candy bar packs a huge caloric punch and won't fill you up; whereas, you may not be able to finish a bowl of less-calorie-dense air-popped popcorn. Which would be a better snack choice?

In one research study of calories versus volume, subjects filled their plates by walking through one side or another of a cafeteria line. They could choose anything they wanted. What they didn't know was that the high-fat version of the food choices was arrayed along one side. On the other side were low-fat versions of the same foods. At the end of the line, plates filled, the researchers measured the total volume of food chosen. Subjects had selected nearly the same volume of food (the food on their plates looked identical), but food chosen from the high-fat side packed a lot more calories. Because we tend to eat the same amount of food regardless of calorie content, the smart plan is to make sure the amount we eat is not packed with calories.

What could be lower in calories than water? But if you buy the myth that you can fill up on water to satisfy food cravings, you probably think a glass of water before or during a meal can stave off hunger.

Not true, says Barbara Rolls, Ph.D., professor and Guthrie chair in nutrition, who heads the Laboratory for the Study of Human Ingestive Behavior at Penn State. Dr. Rolls puts that myth to rest, but has good news too: Eating water-rich foods can lower your calorie intake—and perhaps help you eat less to control your weight.

"The body processes hunger and thirst through different mechanisms," according to Dr. Rolls's research published in *The American Journal of Clinical Nutrition* and in her book *Volumetrics: Feel Full on Fewer Calories.* A beverage will not reduce hunger. But eating water-rich foods such as vegetables, soups and fruits is an effective method for cutting back on calories yet feeling full and satisfied. Also try pasta salad or chili bulked up with veggies and beans, or adding lettuce and tomato to a sandwich.

Feeling full depends on eating a satisfying amount of food. Eat a large bowl of grapes instead of a handful of raisins (same number of calories). One will fill you up while the other will leave you foraging in your refrigerator for more food.

A note about water: You still need your six to eight glasses per day. I suggest you make water your beverage of choice with every meal and between them.

Fad Diets Simply Don't Work

Fad diets can be as tantalizing as the forbidden foods they promise you can eat while losing weight. The currently popular diets work, and you will lose weight—but for all the wrong reasons.

Basic truth #1: You can't follow a fad diet forever

You lose weight on popular high-protein diets, for example, because you're cutting out carbohydrates (potatoes and pasta, breads, fruits and vegetables) that usually make up at least half of your daily calorie intake. But it's not the switch to more protein or busting a "sugar" habit blamed on carbohydrates that causes you to lose weight. It's the drop in the number of calories that carbohydrates usually provide that causes the weight loss.

The diet doctors who write bestselling books don't tell you it's almost impossible to stay on a high-protein, low-carbohydrate diet. The reality is that you can't eat steak and bacon every day or drink the liquid-protein diet drinks that celebrities promote for the rest of your life, nor should you try. When the diet stops, your weight returns with a vengeance because your body quickly replaces lost muscle and fat.

Basic truth #2: On a diet, your body is starving

Eating a lot of protein alone is dangerous and may eventually lead to a condition called ketogenesis in which your body creates toxic levels of ketones that may damage your kidneys beyond repair. Besides causing bad breath and nausea, the ketone production drastically changes your metabolism. You create a condition (much like in famine-stricken people) in which your body will do just the opposite of what you want—instead of processing food normally, everything you eat will fatten you up.

Here's the trap: High-protein diets often aren't high in protein at all. You usually take in too much saturated fat in meats, which may raise cholesterol levels and thus poses an even higher risk for heart problems.

At the other end of the dieting spectrum, just fruit-and-vegetable diets that are extremely low in fat can be dangerous because they often don't supply needed calcium, protein and other nutrients. Besides, vegetarian-type diets don't appeal to everyone. Those trying to keep fat intake below 10 or 20 percent often don't feel satisfied without animal protein and eventually must add lean cuts of meat and fish to fill the nutritional gap. The bottom line is this: Any diet that excludes certain foods is not healthful.

The take-home lesson is that we usually want to eat the same *volume* of food (that's why restrictive diets don't work). Best strategy: Select high-volume foods bulked up with vegetables, for example, and then eat as much food as you normally do. You'll take in fewer calories—yet feel satisfied and "full." So much for cheesecake snack bars. Besides, could one possibly be enough?

Recent research on successful dieters—those who have kept weight off for years—shows that they limit the number of fat calories by paying attention to nutrient density. They have strong *social support* systems, which I know keeps you well. And, just as important, they have incorporated a physical activity program into their lives. You knew I'd work the exercise part in somewhere.

Move It or You Won't Lose

Above all, psychologists say, behavior determines our health. Just knowing what to do doesn't mean you'll do it. Again, it's the old "I know I should lose weight but . . ." rationalization. Successful dieters must actually make behavior changes to add exercise to their lives.

Society, of course, doesn't make exercise easy. Everything we do seems to be designed to be effortless, when in fact we need to expend some of those calories we take in. Those of us who sit in front of computers all day and move a mouse and then go home and sit in front of a TV and move the remote are aware of our low levels of activity.

How Much Should You Weigh?

Another commonly asked question is this: How much should I weigh? The rule of thumb for men is 106 pounds for the first 60 inches of height; then 6 pounds per inch over the first 60 inches. So a reasonable weight for a man at 5 feet, 9 inches in height would be 106 + (9 x 6 inches) or 160 pounds. For women, use 105 pounds for the first 60 inches and 5 pounds per inch after that.

Maintaining a trim weight, ideal for your height and build, can be done. Let me put in a convincing plug for a plant-based diet with meat considered as a side dish. The evidence from the research labs is compelling.

Plant-based foods are rich in vitamins, minerals, fiber and beneficial substances called phytochemicals (*phyto* means plant). All may protect against cancer. In addition, plant-based foods are low in fat and calories. They have the added bonus of helping you maintain a healthy weight.

If a food comes from a plant, eat it often. Fruits, vegetables, legumes, roots, tubers, whole grains and whole-grain products such as wheat bread and cereals should make up the bulk of your diet. They are high in fiber and have a low amount of fats, which are factors in heart disease and possibly for some cancers such as breast, colon and prostate. Legumes include beans, peas and lentils. Common roots and tubers are turnips, beets, potatoes and sweet potatoes.

My colleagues found that quercetin—a plant-based nutrient found most abundantly in apples, onions, tea and red wine—may provide a new method for preventing or treating prostate cancer. Because this cancer usually causes no symptoms, we often don't catch it until it reaches an advanced stage. In a laboratory study here, quercetin reduced or prevented the growth of human prostate cancer cells by blocking activity of androgen hormones. Previous research has linked androgens to prostate cancer's development and progression. Although these results are still early, quercetin may be a potential nonhormonal approach to preventing or treating prostate cancer. This could lend even further credence to the adage about an apple a day.

Or how about a handful of black raspberries a day? Here's another potentially powerful biological weapon for your health. A mix of compounds hiding deep inside the juicy sweetness of black raspberries seemed to hold off tumor formation and progression in rats. Although we'd have to eat several bowls of black raspberries each day to get as much as the rats were fed, it's still sound advice to get your five servings (or more) a day of fruits and vegetables. Strawberries and blueberries also have chemopreventive agents in them, such as anthocyanins, phenols, and vitamins A, C, E, and folic acid. So make one of your daily servings berries.

If you must have food that comes from an animal or is a snack, choose the low-fat version. To cut your fat intake, use low-fat dairy products, choose lean cuts of meat and use vegetable oils. Generally, poultry such as white-meat chicken and turkey are lower in fat than red meats such as beef, pork (which contrary to their marketing is not the "other" white meat) or lamb. But loin cuts of red meats can be low in fat if chosen carefully.

If you must snack, pick those low in fat and choose baked snacks over fried any day.

Let's talk about biochemistry. Some evidence shows that, as we age, chemicals called free radicals are produced by the body. These chemicals in some circumstances can stir things up. They may be able to ignite or start the growth of cancer. These chemicals are thought to possibly have a connection with the development of heart disease, too.

If we can block the development of these free radicals by taking nutritional supplements called antioxidants, there is the hope that the cancer may not occur or that the heart disease might not develop. We're not exactly sure how antioxidants such as vitamin C and vitamin E work, but they may have something to do with slowing the development of cancer and also the aging process.

Again, a tremendous gap exists between the research in the laboratory and the practical application of this research in your life. In general, anti-oxidants obtained from dietary sources (what you eat) are probably better than the antioxidants you buy in a tablet form at Walgreens. At one time, some researchers suggested that vitamin E, for example, would be helpful against heart disease, but that issue is still controversial. Likewise, the role of antioxidants as a way to prevent cancer, while theoretically appealing, has not withstood the scrutiny of rigorously conducted clinical trials.

Low-fat dairy foods such as milk, yogurt and cheese may help control body fat, according to a study presented at the North American Association for the Study of Obesity. Here's how: Mistakenly, people may cut out milk, yogurt and cheese when trying to control weight gain or lose weight. In actuality, low-fat versions of these dairy foods may help control body fat in a well-balanced daily diet. These low-fat foods also may help reduce your risk for developing osteoporosis—a softening of bones that may lead to breaks—because they contain calcium needed to keep bones strong.

Most men don't realize they're at risk for osteoporosis, too. It's no longer a condition reserved just for older women. Drinking milk and doing weight-bearing exercise can greatly increase men's chances of keeping bones strong now and later in life. Like women, men ages nineteen to fifty need at least three 8-ounce glasses of milk or calcium-fortified food such as orange juice each day to help meet the recommended 1,000 milligrams of calcium. Government data confirm that seven out of ten men are not meet-ing these recommendations.

Obesity is a known risk factor for several major types of cancer. Cancers of the breast, the gallbladder, the uterus and the kidney seem to occur in excess among individuals who are over their ideal body weight.

As with all cancers, colon cancer is an example where early detection vir-tually assures cure and a final victory. Although there is ongoing controversy, by increasing the fiber and by decreasing fat in our diet, we can increase our odds of avoiding this problem in the first place. Still, early detection and screening are absolutely vital.

Cancer of the uterus, albeit an infrequent cause of cancer death among women, also seems to be related to obesity and dietary issues. Firm data and solid numbers are elusive, but the drift of evidence suggests that women who can maintain an ideal body weight may well decrease their risk of that cancer as well.

New Diet Approach Makes Sense

Researcher Tracy Sbrocco, Ph.D., at Uniformed Services University is taking a new approach to weight management (not a diet or dieting), and it works. It's a behavioral approach to change. And I have described these points of choice and their role in helping change behavior.

The idea is that you don't worry about weight, but you make very small, permanent changes in your behavior. One week you eat one cookie instead of two if eating cookies is your habit. You park a little farther away from the building at work. Maybe you walk around the block during your lunch break. The following week, you'll walk two blocks. You switch from whole milk to 2 percent. With small steps, you get down to skim milk.

These small changes build slowly over time to become natural, normal behavior. All are designed to increase your energy expenditure or lower your caloric intake. Dr. Sbrocco's work is one of the few approaches to demonstrate sustained weight management over two years or more—which is the key indicator of success.

Life in the Fast-Food Lane

The *Reader's Digest* version of an adequate daily eating guide is this: Multiply your weight in pounds times 10. Therefore, at 180 pounds, you would require approximately 1,800 calories per day. A sedentary person may feel comfortable with this number; conversely, a laborer may require more calories, but at least it's a starting point.

A general guideline would divide these 1,800 calories as follows:

15 to 20 percent protein
55 to 60 percent carbohydrates
25 to 30 percent fat

This means 360 calories of protein, 1,000 calories from carbohydrates and 450 calories from fats. Pay special attention to the fats because saturated fats such as butter and lard are factors in coronary artery disease. Best choices for fats are monounsaturated fats such as olive, canola and peanut oils. Because there are 9 calories per gram of fat, 450 calories $\div$ 9 = 50 grams of fat as the maximum for our 180-pound person. It's best to keep fats at less than 60 grams per day. All this information is on food labels.

If you've ever reached for a food item in the grocery store, turned it over and read the label, chances are you were surprised to see that it was high in fat and put it back. Perhaps you've held two different brands side by side and compared their labels. The standardization in food labeling makes this type of comparison much easier.

After more than six years of such mandatory food labeling, consumers are smarter about high-fat foods on grocery shelves. An economist at Cornell University found that sales of high-fat salad dressings significantly dropped after mandatory food labeling—potentially evidence that the labels really are influencing the sales of other high-fat foods as well.

Are you always on the go? Too often, dinner is a grab-and-dash(board) affair. Eating healthfully in the fast-food lane can be done. It's all part of that balance between calories and fat and protein and depends, of course, on what else you've eaten that day. Although these foods don't come with easy-to-consult food labels, you can find out what's in them. Most fast-food chains publish their menu contents and break down the number of calories and fat grams. Ask for a brochure next time you drive through or check out nutritional information on the Internet; here are some helpful places to "drive" by:

www.mcdonalds.com
www.burgerking.com
www.arbys.com
www.tacobell.com

Many of us have little understanding of grams of fat per serving, despite the easier-to-read food labeling, so let's look at some real examples.

- Looks are deceiving. Sometimes the fast-food salad is not the best choice. For example, at McDonald's, the Grilled Chicken Caesar Salad, just 100 calories and 2.5 grams of fat, sounds attractive, but add a salad dressing such as ranch (170 calories, 18 grams of fat) and you're better off with a hamburger. However, McDonald's offers fat-free herb vinaigrette for the salad dressing, and that's just 35 calories and no fat.

- At McDonald's, you can load up on a Big Mac's 590 calories and 34 grams of fat or instead choose a hamburger with 280 calories and 10 grams of fat. Heck, **two** hamburgers still have less fat and fewer calories than **one** Big Mac. A better choice, however, would be the Chicken McGrill's 300 calories and 6 fat grams.

- At Burger King, you can have it their way, a double Whopper with cheese, and 1,150 calories and 76 grams of fat later, you've just eaten enough for two people. Rein in your appetite and go for the single Whopper, yet you're still getting 760 calories and 46 grams of fat. Ask for it your way (without mayonnaise), and you drop to 600 calories and 28 grams of fat. Still not acceptable. The hamburger, by contrast, is 310 calories and 13 grams of fat. Keep driving.

- Arby's Market Fresh Sandwiches look healthful and delicious. They are. Delicious. But the calorie ranges are between 730 and 880 per sandwich with fat grams 33 to 44. That honey-wheat bread may provide needed fiber, but what's between the slices could put you in an ambulance. The regular roast beef sandwich contains 350 calories and 16 fat grams, by comparison—still not a smart choice too often.

So can you eat healthfully in the fast-food lane? Yes, carefully:

- Supersized is out. Order individually. Super meals are only super deals if you want high calories and fat content.
- Order the single or even remove the hamburger or discard the bun.
- Get low-fat milk or water instead of a soft drink.
- The salad is usually a better choice. But select your dressing carefully or use only part of the dressing. Dip your fork in the dressing on the side, then stab your lettuce.
- Eat prudently the rest of the day.

Dining out poses its own challenges when you've got the menu propped in front of you. Everything sounds great, and you're about to make a decision based on your level of hunger, which is probably high because that's why you're sitting in a restaurant. Many restaurants these days like to win you over with huge quantities. If you see patrons walking away with white Styrofoam boxes, you can guess the portion size is rather large.

Your best bet is to stick to baked or grilled or broiled items, not fried. Order sauce on the side or season your pasta or fish or salad with fresh lemon. Salad dressing should be ordered on the side. Instead of butter and sour cream on that baked potato, try salsa or low-fat cottage cheese.

Upscale restaurants may allow you to share an entrée and simply charge you for "another plate." It's worth the money, and you won't go away hungry.

Or ask your server to put half of your meal in a "doggy bag" (who are we kidding, the dog never sees this stuff) in the kitchen before serving you. What you don't see, you won't miss, and then you'll have a nice white box to take home for tomorrow. It's also quite acceptable to ask for a smaller portion. I can't imagine a restaurant that wouldn't accommodate this request.

ARE WE MEN AND WOMEN, OR ARE WE MICE?

Let me pose this question: We know what's good for us, so why don't we follow it? To answer this question, I turn to the experts. Rats. They eat anything, right?

A study was conducted in Philadelphia and published in the *American Journal of Physiology* to measure whether test animals who were allowed to choose from containers filled with different life-sustaining nutrients would eat from each one and choose a balanced diet with all necessary nutrients. The thinking is that if rats can do it, so can humans. Teenagers might have been another group to test, but we already know they don't eat a balanced diet.

Researchers ended the test early because four of seven rats given extra cups of carbohydrates and three of the seven given additional fat ate so little protein they died—even though protein was freely available to them. Switch gears now and look at what your children see (or what you see) when you open the refrigerator door. The good stuff is there, just like it was for the rats, but do you and your kids make selections like the rats? The chips, the dip, soft drinks, ice cream, high-fat prepared foods? What about the apples, orange juice and cottage cheese?

A similar test was done with drinks. New batches of test rats were put into three groups. One group received just water. The second received five bottles of water and one bottle of sucrose (it's sugar, so think of this as the rat version of Coke). The third received one bottle of water and five bottles of sucrose. The researchers found that the rats with five bottles of sucrose drank a ton of it, and at the same time ate much less, but gained more weight as a result of the added sugar intake. All rats given access to sucrose gained weight.

(continued on following page)

Our take-home lesson is that we should not have soft drinks readily available for our children and ourselves. We'll drink it. And, like the rats, we'll gain weight.

If you think about it, just as my colleagues who conducted these rat studies have, maybe the causes for the obesity epidemic lie not in our genetic makeup, hormonal differences or body weight after all, even though we'd like to think we can place blame on things we can't control. The causes may have much more to do with the availability of food—portion size, what's on sale at the grocery store, menu items in school and work cafeterias, what activities our kids do (and don't do) after school, and selections in the ever-present vending machines.

Let's Put the Grocery Cart Before The . . .*

Every time you sit down to a meal, you may increase or decrease your risk of getting cancer. In fact, the National Cancer Institute estimates that if everyone ate right, cancer deaths would be reduced by a third. But determining what is "right" for you is different from what is right for me. And therein lies the problem.

Whether you're eating at home, dining while driving, ordering out in restaurants or grabbing take-away foods to eat at the office, every meal offers a chance to make healthy choices. But the place we make the most food choices is actually in the grocery store.

Supermarket savvy

Make a list, check it twice. Before you even walk inside the supermarket, always make a list. If you don't, you will buy stuff you never dreamed you'd have in your cart. At the same time, never go shopping when you're hungry because you'll sample and buy food you had no intention of eating. I'm guilty of that. I find myself picking up those little food samples, such as pizza, which I'd never eat in a million years.

But before you even head to the grocery store, sit down and plan out a

* This section was developed in consultation with Peggy Menzel, R.D.

week's worth of menus. This gets easier the more you do it. Focus on what to have for the main item for the meal. For example, Monday will be chicken, then decide what goes with that. Salad and baked potatoes. Tuesday will be fish. Wednesday is a meatless day. Thursday is hamburgers. Fish again on Friday, and Saturday, roast pork. Then work on what you want to add to those meals.

Change your thinking a little by making meat the accompaniment to the meal—almost a side dish. Make no more than three to four ounces of meat per person, if you choose to serve meat, which we don't. That's about the size of a deck of cards, and it's a good "deal." An ideal meal would be a boneless, skinless chicken breast; a small salad with green leafy lettuce and tomatoes, carrots and cucumber; a cup of steamed broccoli; and a small-to-medium baked potato (about the size of a tennis ball).

Let's talk about salad dressing. A lot of people don't like the taste of the low-fat dressings. Make your own with oil and vinegar and a little blue cheese. But here's the best technique. Put the dressing on the side and dip your fork in the dressing first, then stab the vegetables. It's amazing how much less you'll use. So when you order out, request your dressings and sauces on the side and use this technique. That way, you have total control over what you put on your food and in your mouth.

For dessert, how about a nice bowl of fresh cut fruit salad, nothing on it? Or spoon some low-fat or nonfat vanilla yogurt over the fruit or mix it all together.

Cooking is becoming a lost art. No one wants to do much cooking, which is why we turn to convenience foods and fast foods. They're quick and sometimes acceptable for an occasional meal. Try not to get into the habit of making a stop at KFC part of your standard fare. You can make better soup than Campbell's and a better dinner than Swanson. Plan menus and shop accordingly.

Ready, set, shop

Shop the perimeter. As your menus come together, your list of ingredients will be building. You'll find that most of the better choices are found around the perimeter of the store. The fresh fruits and vegetables, bakery, meats and dairy are usually arranged around the outside, while the more processed foods are in the center aisles and frozen cases. Your plan is to shop the perimeter and venture into the center only as needed. It's a jungle in there!

If you're like most American shoppers, you'll spend an average of twenty-two minutes shopping, and you'll make about two trips to a grocery store each week, according to Phil Lempert, who studies our shopping habits at *www.supermarketguru.com*. You'll spend a total of ninety-one dollars, and a third of your purchases will be made on impulse.

So let's go shopping together here, virtually. I'll help you make the most of your twenty-two minutes.

Make bright choices in the fruits and vegetables section

Spend the majority of your twenty-two minutes among the fruits and vegetables. Pick out ripe or ripening produce. Your selection will depend on the season, of course, and where you live. In summer, you'll find more melons and better grapes and mangoes. Take advantage of this variety in the summer.

Go for pigment. Choose as many different brilliantly colored fruits as you can, such as strawberries, blueberries, bananas, oranges, apples and melons.

Your best choices among the vegetables are dark green leafy ones (such as romaine, red leaf lettuce or spinach—not iceberg lettuce). Select the colorful pigments of carrots, broccoli, peppers (green, red and orange), cauliflower, green beans, asparagus and more. When forced to choose, buy less ripe rather than too ripe.

Why go for color? All these foods contain phytochemicals (the good stuff from plants), antioxidants and fiber.

The surprising truth about organic foods

Is organic better? Organic simply means the fruits and vegetables were grown without pesticides. This may be important to you if you eat the peel on fruits such as apples. And certainly it's hard to avoid eating the peel on grapes.

I often don't choose organic produce because, frankly, it looks as if it's been sitting there for three weeks. I hate to pay as much or more and then have it go bad (though I've found bagged organic lettuce is fine). I wash, rinse and dry my fruits and veggies to remove any residue. Water works just as well as any special sprays. The important thing is to dry the fruit. Then water won't sit in the bottom of the bowl and cause the produce to go bad. I let everything ripen on the kitchen counter. Some items such as avocados and pears do well ripening in a plain brown-paper bag.

What if you've never tried a kumquat or an ugli fruit and you're unsure if it's ripe or how to cut and cook it. Try something novel when dining out or at somebody's house before you buy. If you're not sure you'll like it, see if you can buy half rather than a whole. For recipes, consult basic cookbooks, go online or check your library for books that will help you cook some of these unknown delicacies in small quantities. Many supermarkets have shopper's guides on display in the produce department for sale or for information. And, of course, you can ask the produce manager. These experts can help choose the ripest cantaloupe in the bunch or give you pointers on pomegranates and kiwifruit. They can even describe the taste. Don't be surprised if the manager cuts one for you to taste.

When you buy fresh fruit, keep it on the counter in a nice pretty bowl. Otherwise, you won't see your produce in the refrigerator until it's time to throw it away when it withers in the crisper. If you don't see it, you won't eat it. But if a fresh bunch of green grapes or a bright yellow banana is calling your name from the countertop, chances are you'll grab it and go.

Freeze those luscious and abundant grapes for a fun summer treat. Stick peeled bananas onto Popsicle sticks and freeze. Fruit that gets too ripe can be frozen and plopped into smoothies later. (Peel and cut up the bananas first.)

Ripe vegetables can be put in other dishes, such as casseroles and homemade soup. If your family hates cabbage, put it into something they like, such as minestrone soup. The picky eaters are less likely to pick it out.

Experiment with different seasonings. Lemon juice or balsamic vinegar on broccoli may become a favorite in lieu of a heavy cheese sauce or butter. Jazz things up with fresh ground black pepper, fresh herbs and spices.

Frozen fruits are fine, but . . . make sure the fruit wasn't frozen along with a lot of sugar. Check the label. Look for sugar among the top three ingredients. Sugar can often be disguised as fructose or sucrose, so avoid the "-ose" endings. Your prospects for canned fruit are much better. Look for fruit packed in its own juice or water or light syrup. Avoid anything labeled with heavy syrup.

I prefer frozen vegetables over canned. Especially if you're cooking for one, it's sure easier to make a smaller portion from a frozen box of peas. Canned vegetables are a last resort. Many are high in salt (the label will call it sodium), and unsalted canned vegetables usually taste awful. Plus they're often more expensive.

Juices are controversial. You can get your daily servings this way, but limit your consumption of 100 percent fruit juice to just one to two servings (and that's just a half-cup per serving). You can add extra calories if you drink more, plus you'll miss the fiber and nutrients from whole fresh fruit.

When it comes to meat, think small

Continuing around the perimeter of your grocery store, you'll get to the meat section. Some of us choose not to eat meat for various reasons. This is an individual decision. But if you choose to eat meat, some tips will help you use the meat counter to your advantage.

Think small. Think about eating red meat only two or three times a week. The Mediterranean food guide pyramid, based on the heart-healthy diet of our friends in the Greek Islands, puts meat almost in the same category as sweets—limited amounts, not every day. Instead of red meat or the "other" white meat (pork), try fish, poultry or go meatless. When you choose to have meat, I encourage you to limit portion size to a deck of cards (a single deck!). Women can be guided by the rule of thumb of no more than five ounces per day; men about six ounces. That deck of cards is about three ounces.

So you can see that a pound of ground beef, with the lowest possible fat content, at sixteen ounces will go a long way. If you choose not to buy the 95 percent lean burger, then buy the higher-fat-content meat, cook it, and then drain it well in a colander and even rinse it with water to remove fat. The flavor will depend on the seasonings you put into it.

Use ground turkey in place of ground beef, but check your labels; you want ground white turkey meat, not the dark meat or the skin.

You may have heard about and even tried TVP. That's texturized vegetable protein, by any other name, soy protein (plant-based). These meat substitutes are virtually indistinguishable if you use them in chili or lasagna, but it may take getting used to if you dress it up with a bun as a hamburger substitute.

When you select meats, go for cuts with the word *loin* in them. These are lean cuts, contain less saturated fat (the bad stuff), and the butchers have probably trimmed off all visible fat. If they haven't, you can.

Chicken is amazingly versatile. A three-pound package of boneless, skinless breasts can feed a family of four until the next millennium. But take the skin off any chicken you buy before you cook it. If you insist, cook with the skin on to keep the chicken more moist, but take the skin off before you eat it—and don't eat the skin.

Got milk?

Rounding the corner to the dairy aisle, still along the perimeter of the grocery store, you'll want to pick up skim milk. Actually 1 percent milk is fine, too. Watch the labels on yogurt to make sure you get the low-fat or fat-free varieties. Eating regular yogurt is like eating a dish of ice cream. Low-fat or fat-free yogurt acts like a dessert without the guilt. Try it on top of angel food cake or mix it with your breakfast cereal.

Flour power

You may have to venture inside the aisles to get to the bread. Because we're in the North Country, we get a wonderful loaf of bread from the Manitowoc Ovens in Wisconsin. It has five grams of fiber per slice (that's a lot, and that's what bread is for). Compare that with a half to two grams per slice for regular "store-bought" breads. You'll get ten grams, of course, with a sandwich, which is more fiber than most people get in a day, but need. In fact, we need 25 to 35 grams every day.

If you can find bread listed as having two or more grams per slice, buy it. Your store should have some excellent local brands. But the most important ingredient listed on the label is the flour itself. You want "100 percent whole-wheat flour" listed as the first ingredient on the label. If it's not, put the loaf back and keep reading labels until you find those four magic words. Breads calling themselves wheat bread or whole wheat or whole grain or seven- or twelve-grain may not be the real deal and may just be the equivalent of plain white bread that's brown. The label tells the whole truth and nothing but.

Maybe you don't like wheat bread or your family refuses to eat it. Try a sandwich with one slice of whole wheat and one slice of white. But if you lose this battle, just make sure whatever you put between the slices is healthy stuff.

Deli delights

Can you make it past the deli without stopping for the free samples? Actually, the deli case may have some good choices, such as lean cuts of turkey and roast beef. Stay away from processed meats such as salami or bologna. Avoid the fried chicken, but the roast chicken is usually delicious (without the skin).

Add some cheeses to your meats by selecting those made with part skim milk, such as mozzarella.

Fresh deli salads are tempting, but avoid those made with mayonnaise bases, such as the potato and macaroni salads. And the marshmallow-whipped-cream salads are also to be avoided. If you have the deli make you a sandwich, opt for mustard not mayo, or select light mayo.

Tempting bargains

Watch those end caps. These are the ends of the grocery aisles where the real bargains lurk. If you see something on sale, you can think of all kinds of reasons to load up your cart with half-price Halloween candy and the two-for-one ice cream specials. If you're not careful, you'll buy the Brooklyn Bridge, too. You don't need an excuse to cruise right on by the specials; you have your list. Stick to it.

Except when it's fresh apples or canned peaches. These are harmless and helpful menu items. But leave behind the crackers or cookies and chips you think you need because the grandkids are coming in three months. You can always put them on your list for next time.

By the time you steer your healthfully filled cart into the checkout lane, you won't be lured by the tabloids hyping a "diet of the day" anymore. You won't have to wonder what's for dinner because you will have stocked up for the next several days. And you won't be tempted to stop at a fast-food or convenience store for cardiac cruise missiles.

Experts help choose the foods you use

Many of us struggle with food and food issues. Because Peggy is a registered dietitian, I can work closely with my own food consultant. But I do recommend that you arrange to meet with a registered dietitian (R.D.), especially to design a heart-healthy eating plan or if you are managing other chronic conditions such as diabetes.

Talk with your doctor about a referral. Many R.D.s work through hospitals, clinics and private practice. You are seeking the credential of "R.D.," and not nutritionist or personal trainer or something else. This is specific and highly specialized training. Others who pretend to understand nutrition may try to sell you all kinds of unneeded and perhaps dangerous dietary supplements. Now, many states require the credential of L.D. (licensed dietitian) in addition to the R.D. degree.

Expect to sit down with the R.D. and discuss your dietary history. This would include your lifestyle (eating on the run, business trips, cooking for kids, cooking for one), your health habits (exercise), whether you travel or work night shifts, and how often you might eat out. The R.D. will want to know if you like to cook or never cook. You may be asked to keep a food diary for a week or so.

From this thorough dietary and lifestyle history, the R.D. will help you develop an individual program. Together you can figure out the number of calories you need every day. You can set goals for weight loss, for lowering cholesterol, for controlling blood glucose levels, for lowering blood pressure. And you'll decide what your priorities are and what to do first. You won't want to move too quickly or too drastically. You want to make lifelong lifestyle changes.

Many times, if you begin an exercise program first and watch your caloric intake, the weight will take care of itself, if weight loss is your goal. A qualified R.D. will help you set a realistic weight-loss goal. Toss out those jeans from high school you wish you still fit into—those outrageous expectations will only defeat you.

Is one-a-day enough or even necessary?

Now let me say that I'm not opposed to vitamins, but you don't need to overdo it. Everything you need, you can get from food. But a one-a-day multivitamin for added assurance is usually fine for most people. Your doctor may suggest particular supplements for you. But it's my experience that some people who take vitamins often have no idea why or how much they should take and what the supplements are supposed to be doing.

My Thoughts . . .

We really do become what we eat. For me, I do all I can to shift the odds in my favor. In fact, I won't let the airlines dictate what they can serve me. I order a low-fat meal when I make my flight reservations or bring my own healthier snacks. Of course, I'm not naive. And I do not believe for a moment that I can avoid cancer or heart disease altogether, but I do believe that I can have a better hand to play if I stay in charge. So can you.

Only you are responsible for what you're putting into your mouth. Because there is no question that excess body weight is responsible for heart disease and some cancers, you can use the tips here to eat defensively for your good health.

5

Deal with Reasonable Chaos and Gain Strength Through Stress

All the resources we need are in the mind.

—Theodore Roosevelt

It used to be, if you worked hard, showed up and did your job, your employer would take care of you. That was then. Working Americans now feel disposable and replaceable. And those entering the workforce today can anticipate a minimum of five career shifts in their professional lifetimes—maybe more.

We counsel high school and college students about portable skills and marketable traits as they put together their portfolios of values and interests. These will be the tools that serve them in their quest and will be there when they need to bounce back as they bounce from job to job in today's marketplace.

Job security? Gone. Mergers, acquisitions, consolidations, restructuring and downsizing have created a new Willy Loman—it's all *About Schmidt* and Jack Nicholson's dead-on portrayal of what may lie ahead for many Americans when released from the corporate cocoon. We witness the death of this salesman over and over again. Long-term employment is a phenomenon of the past. It is unlikely that anyone will spend an entire career under one corporate umbrella anymore. Many corporate umbrellas are imploding under their own ineptitude, dumping disenfranchised employees and disgruntled stockholders. And regardless of your career status, the skills required to maintain your current position will be obsolete in five to seven years.

About 70 percent of working people feel "used up" at day's end, and half describe themselves as "highly stressed." More than 25 percent of us—right now—have stress-induced illnesses.

Stress can suppress your immune system, making you susceptible to infectious diseases—viruses such as flu or bacterial infections such as tuberculosis. Stress causes the heart to beat quicker, which makes you vulnerable to chest pain (angina) and irregular heart rhythms. Stress may even lead to heart attack or stroke.

Stress is indeed a health issue, and who isn't stressed today?

My point? The workplace is changing. These profound changes affect our health, and the workplace is where the effects of health are so obvious. Today's workforce is mobile. Your current employer has little vested interest in keeping you healthy over the long-term so you'll live longer and healthier because, chances are, you won't be working at that company in your later years when all the prevention measures you could take now start to pay off in terms of longevity. In fact, you may be a liability to your employer if you collect on retirement plans or remain on a company's health insurance plan because you're living longer and healthier. They'd rather you didn't collect your gold watch and full pension.

Work itself contributes to stress. Service-with-a-smile takes a toll. Those of you engaged in "emotional labor" know all too well the incredible strains on your mental and physical abilities. Emotional labor refers to the process of controlling emotions that is required by service workers such as retail clerks, secretaries, flight attendants and others who are expected to cope with sometimes difficult customers and clients. Difficult interactions can result in negative mental and physical health, says a Penn State researcher in the *Journal of Occupational Health Psychology*.

"Service with a smile, especially when mandated by a company, may be pleasing to the customer, but at the same time, it may be emotionally and physically stressful for the employee, especially if forced or insincere," said Alicia A. Grandey, assistant professor of industrial and organizational psychology. "Job stress does more than cause absenteeism, decreased productivity, fatigue and burnout. The physiological bottling-up of emotions taxes the body over time by overworking the cardiovascular and nervous systems, and weakening the immune system."

If you're in one of these service-with-a-smile positions—and difficult customers start to get to you—learn to redirect your emotional response. I encourage you to take a brief walk, begin deep-breathing exercises or try internal self-talk that allows you to reappraise a bad experience with a customer—especially if your employer doesn't have similar debriefing strategies.

What's your alternative? A job with few responsibilities and no customer contact? Mindless jobs, on one hand, might sound attractive to stressed-out, battle-worn workers. But think again. Working Americans with little opportunity for decision making die earlier than those with more flexibility, even if those flexible jobs are also high-stress positions, according to a study out of the University of Texas.

"The lack of control a person had in his or her job substantially increased the hazard of death," said Benjamin C. Amick III, Ph.D., who led the research team. They found that workers with little control in their jobs were 43 to 50 percent more likely to die during a period of five to ten years than workers who had high-stress jobs but more decision-making responsibilities.

Meaningfulness of work, then, like meaningfulness in life can make a difference in your health. In the 1940s, an Austrian-born psychiatrist, Dr. Viktor Frankl, was imprisoned in a concentration camp during the Holocaust. He survived an incredibly soul-shredding experience and tried to discern why some survived and some died. He made the observation that prisoners who had a reason to live, who had a "why" to live, somehow crafted the "how" to live. In other words, *meaning* and *purpose* somehow gave them the will to survive.

How Do We Find Meaning and Purpose in What We Do?

There are no easy answers, but the long-term survivors in science, in business and in a variety of professions seem to have the following characteristics, and I discuss this in more detail in the last chapter of this book:

- Survivors have their health. If our health goes south, nothing else matters. Just think about the last time you had surgery, the flu, an infection or an injury. The last thing you thought about was your 401(k), your investment portfolio or your projects at work. And those who lose their health can still maintain a sense of "wellness." Think about it. "Health" and "wellness" are two quite different states. For example, someone with a major disability may not be physically healthy but is certainly "well" in a powerful sense. Whereas an Olympic athlete—the epitome of physical health—could be a child abuser and not "well" at all.

- Survivors have a sense of community, a sense of connectedness. They somehow bond with colleagues, and a common task can generate a communal energy, which is greater than any one individual can generate.
- Survivors always have a sense of challenge; they never become complacent. I became intrigued with entertainers Siegfried and Roy, for example. I asked them how they can perform the same Las Vegas show thousands of times—a grueling schedule physically and mentally. Each responded that he always tries to make it perfect—fully recognizing that the show can never be perfect. This keeps them going night after night, performance after performance, week after week, because they love what they do.
- Survivors always look for new challenges and new opportunities and face each day as a gift and as a promise.

Many years ago, Eleanor Roosevelt made the comment that the future belongs to those who believe in the beauty of their dreams. The individuals who are most prepared to face the future are those who create the future rather than waiting for life to simply happen to them, like a cork adrift on the sea subject to the wind, waves and current.

HOW DOES YOUR BODY SAY "I'M STRESSED"?

Keeping your internal stress a secret is not easy. Stressed-out people do a number of incredibly annoying things with their bodies. Business communications expert Barbara Pachter points out that it's what you **don't** say that says a lot about you. She has listed the top ten non-verbal cues that say "I'm stressed" in her book *The Power of Positive Confrontation:*

1. Point finger at others
2. Stick out tongue/lick lips when speaking
3. Wring their hands
4. Sway
5. Use very stern facial expression
6. Use too broad or no gestures at all/hands on hips
7. Pound fist
8. Tap foot when seated
9. Look at floor when speaking
10. Play with change in pocket

Check these behaviors at your next employee meeting and see if you can spot who's stressed. Let's hope it's not you.

It's About Time

Manage your time as if your life depended on it . . . because it does.
—Robert S. Eliot, M.D.

These days, time management is not optional. Without it, stress levels would really be out of control. The average working American is putting in fifty-hour weeks and has become enslaved by a fiberoptic noose. Yet none of these so-called labor-saving devices—computer, fax, cell phone, personal digital assistant, e-mail—has really saved any time whatsoever. Time has become a noose around our collective necks. Laboratory animals bombarded by uncontrollable stimuli like this are not happy campers. And neither are we.

A Pitney Bowes survey counted 190 messages every working day for the average person. These interruptions included telephone calls, voice mails, electronic planner messages, beepers, e-mail messages—and all required a response. No wonder we're stressed and can't get anything done.

If we permit interruptions, we're making one of the five worst mistakes of time management. The other four mistakes of time management are these:

- Spending time on issues that are not your priority
- Underestimating the time a task consumes—nothing is simple
- Saying "yes" without thinking
- Not asking for help

One of the most important times in time management (and stress reduction) is what I call the psychological "moat." This is a buffer of time between commitments. Transition time, in other words. This is the zone in which we switch gears to psychologically prepare for the next challenge. But how many of us grab files and dash into meetings or to the next customer, without readying our minds for the next mental challenge? We certainly wouldn't show up for the tennis or golf match of our lifetime just a few minutes before the event.

One place to win the time-management battle is the dreaded "meeting." Realistically, most meetings are held for historical or informational purposes only. Little is accomplished. A Harvard Business School study says 90 percent of meetings accomplish very little. Meanwhile, you're sitting there, and time is tick, tick, ticking away. If you're in a position to make it happen, insist on an agenda and prompt start and stop times. Otherwise, you're wasting everyone's time.

Delegation is another winner in the time-management equation. No one individual can meet the needs of an organization. Each of us at the start of the day has so many units of energy. We must decide how to prioritize time and talents, or someone else will. Constructive delegation of responsibility frees us to focus on important tasks and empowers others.

You may have heard this story or read a forwarded version of this unattributed Internet wisdom, but indulge me as I retell it in my own way.

When is your jar full?

A philosophy professor stood before the class with a large empty mayonnaise jar and proceeded to fill it with large rocks. He then asked students if the jar was full. They agreed it was.

So the professor picked up a box of pebbles and poured them into the jar. He shook the jar lightly. The pebbles, of course, rolled into the open areas between the rocks.

"Is the jar full now?" he asked.

The students agreed the jar was full. The professor picked up a box of sand and poured it into the jar. Of course, the sand filled up everything else.

"Now," said the professor, "I want you to recognize that this is your life. The rocks are the important things—your family, your partner, your health, your children—things that if everything else was lost and only they remained, your life would still be full.

"The pebbles are the other things that matter, like your job, your house, your car," he said.

"The sand is everything else. The small stuff."

Because this was a philosophy class, the professor went on to explain: "If you put the sand into the jar first, there is no room for the pebbles or the rocks. The same goes for your life. If you spend all your time and energy on the small stuff, you will never have room for the things that are important to you. Pay attention to the things that are critical to your happiness. Play with your children. Take time to get medical checkups. Take your partner out dancing. There will always be time to go to work, clean the house, give a dinner party and fix the disposal. Take care of the rocks first—the things that really matter. Set your priorities. The rest is just sand."

Examine what you have in your mayonnaise jar. Are you sweating the pebbles—the small stuff—or the sand? Or do you make time to put the rocks in first?

Of course, this delightful (albeit apocryphal) story came over the Internet, and it continues. A student took the jar, which all had agreed was quite full, and poured a glass of beer into it. The moral is that there's always room for beer, but this is a book about prevention and the chapter that covers alcohol use is just ahead!

I divide time (the rocks, pebbles and sand of life) into the following types:

- **Prime time.** These are those hours (or minutes) of the day when your energy can be focused like a heat-seeking missile. No interruptions. If you're working, this is the work time when you're at your peak. For me, it's the early morning hours. Tackle your hardest work when you are the sharpest. Your enthusiasm during this time has a targeted velocity. Guard this time with the intensity of a Rottweiler. Do not give it away. This is your hour of power.
- **Brain-stem time.** Use this for mechanical, mundane chores such as sorting out junk mail, signing routine correspondence and minding other mindless burdens that can be effectively dispatched during this time.
- **Away time.** These are precious occasions when we are physically removed from the arena and can direct our energies to tasks of renewal. We golf, garden, run, paint—these activities revive body and soul. Away time allows us to remove the yoke for a short time and know that we do not have to save the world—at least for today. In other words, leave the laptop at home, or you might as well be at the office. Sad but true, a laptop ad in *The Wall Street Journal* says it well: "The good news is that you're always connected to the office. The bad news is that you are always connected to the office."

In planning your time, it's preferable to avoid time leaks. Phone calls, e-mail and faxes can quickly become enormous time-wasters and block your coronary arteries. They do not save time. Try to handle routine inquiries between specific hours. Return messages just before lunch and just before you leave for the day. Research has shown that messages responded to at these times are typically shorter. Keep pen in hand to complete uncomplicated paperwork so that time spent waiting on hold or waiting for a Web page to download is not completely wasted.

What I do

I'm a list maker. I plan the week, not just the day. And I plan *away time* for each day or evening. If I write down the tasks, I greatly increase the chance they'll get done. And it puts me in the driver's seat. Checking things off my list is empowering. Try it.

CREATE YOUR PSYCHOLOGICAL MOAT

1. **Do not spend time on issues that are not your priority.** That means making a list in the morning or in the prior evening so you can do what is important to you that day. Otherwise, your work culture will siphon off your time and you'll go home feeling frustrated and unfulfilled.

2. **Nothing is simple.** Everything takes three times longer than expected, so never underestimate the time something will take.

3. **If you say "yes" to interruptions, you are giving away a piece of your soul.** Turning off the pager, turning off the e-mail and turning off your computer may help save your life.

4. **If you continually say "yes" to everything, you in effect are saying "yes" to nothing.** We have so many units of energy in the morning and if we do not determine how we use them, they will quickly evaporate like the early morning dew.

Our response to stress is highly individual. But generally it's like a football player who has repetitive trauma in the game. One hit and he'll survive. But add up week after week of hits in a season, and he'll be hurting. He won't be able to handle it anymore.

Are you taking too many hits? Feeling too stressed? Here are five telltale signs:

1. You feel irritable.
2. You have sleep problems (you're either sleepy all the time or can't sleep).
3. You experience no joy.
4. You develop a severe loss of appetite, or you can't stop eating.
5. You have trouble with relationships and no longer get along well with friends and family members.

Don't Like the Movie? Rewrite the Script

It's all about attitude. Your outlook on life, in fact, not only may help you live longer, but it appears to have an impact on your quality of life. Those of us who see the glass half-full (the optimists) report a higher level of physical and mental functioning than those who see the glass half-empty and don't look on the bright side of life (the pessimists). One of my colleagues has looked at the half-full glass, and his research is showing that outlook on life may help extend it.

"The wellness of being is not just physical, but attitudinal," said Toshihiko Maruta, M.D., lead author of the study published in *Mayo Clinic Proceedings*. "How you perceive what goes on around you and how you interpret it may have an impact on your longevity, and it could affect the quality of your later years."

Study participants were surveyed in the 1960s with a personality test and again thirty years later. This is one of the first studies to report the long-term health effects of self-reported outlook.

This study shows that if we can see a light at the end of the tunnel, we can see a positive good regardless of the circumstances. There's no question that to some extent we can determine our reality. We can learn to focus on what we have rather than on what we don't have.

For my cancer patients, this is rock solid. I can tell who's an optimist, and who is not, the moment I walk into the exam room. The distinction is startling.

Even with heart disease, a sense of optimism seems to protect health. Based on a scoring system that placed a group of men on a scale from pessimist to optimist, each step up the scale toward optimism decreased their risk of coronary heart disease. The most optimistic men had a risk of heart disease less than half of that for the most grouchy of the old men, according to a study headed by a Harvard researcher in the journal *Psychosomatic Medicine*.

The men were drawn from a group of veterans in their sixties who were followed for an average of ten years. The researchers suggest that the protective effects of optimism may be, in part, caused by lower stress, which has been shown to decrease heart-disease risk. Also, the optimists in the study were more likely to engage in health-promoting activities such as exercise and not be smokers.

The researchers caution that the results are specific only to the study group, but let's be optimistic and say that stress management and having a healthy outlook on life certainly can't hurt.

But simple, cost-effective treatment can help people with diabetes control blood sugar, and I'm not talking about insulin shots. It's about stress management.

A smile a day can keep the doctor away, in certain circumstances. Stress can increase glucose levels in people with diabetes, making them more susceptible to long-term physical complications such as eye, kidney or nerve disorders. In the short term, uncontrolled stress may lead to the release of hormones that activate the fight-or-flight response, dumping glucose into the bloodstream—which poses a health threat for someone with diabetes.

Participants in a research study at Duke University Medical Center with type 2 diabetes were taught how to identify everyday life stressors and how to respond to them with such techniques as progressive muscle relaxation, mental imagery and breathing exercises.

The Duke researchers were able to show that these stress-management techniques, when added to standard care, helped reduce glucose levels, as much as might be expected with control drugs alone. The results were published in the journal *Diabetes Care*.

The only way to survive our stressful existence is to recognize that we have choices and options in the way we live and respond to stress. Let me offer fifteen proven ways to reduce stress:

1. Simplify your life. Cut out some activities or delegate tasks. Use the extra time to relax—use such exercises as controlling your breathing, clearing your mind and relaxing your muscles.
2. View negative situations as positive and a chance to improve your life.
3. Use humor to reduce or relieve tension.
4. Exercise. It relieves tension and provides a "time out" from stressful situations.
5. Go to bed earlier. More sleep makes you stronger and more able to handle day-to-day life.
6. Reduce or eliminate caffeine. Caffeine is a stimulant.
7. Get a massage.
8. Keep a stress journal. Track what "sets you off" and learn to prioritize tasks. Do what is most important first.
9. Enjoy yourself. Read a good book or see an uplifting movie.

10. Take a hot bath.
11. Call a friend and strengthen or establish a support network. Make the most of friends and family.
12. Set aside personal time. Limit time spent with "negative" people.
13. Hug your family and friends and pets.
14. Do volunteer work or start a hobby.
15. Take a vacation. Take a day or longer to rejuvenate yourself.

These quick, simple techniques to manage stress can often do more than my colleagues and I can with medication.

Although there is little credible evidence that stress causes cancer, stress certainly can make your life miserable. It seems most reasonable to make all appropriate efforts to keep life at a reasonable level of chaos.

Gain Strength Through Stress

You can harness stress and turn it around. In other words, you can gain strength through stress. My colleague, the late Robert Eliot, M.D., a cardiologist, was among the first to clearly recognize that there is a solid connection between attitude, disposition and susceptibility to disease. Dr. Eliot documented that the mind–body connection is indisputable, and our attitudes and our outlook have a clear bearing on the occurrence of illness.

- He pointed out unmistakably that many heart attacks occur on a Monday morning. Even his own.
- Accountants and those in related professions are at especially high stress during the first quarter of the year preparing for income taxes—all leading up to April 15.
- Longshoremen in San Francisco who were physically working on the docks had a much lower rate of heart disease than the managers who were not physically active but who were under tremendous stress.

Dr. Eliot was a prominent cardiologist in Omaha who had a busy practice and was an acknowledged expert in the management of heart disease. His book *From Stress to Strength: How to Lighten Your Load and Save Your Life* focuses on the importance of nutrition, exercise, time management and identifying our stresses and strengths. He was a pioneer in his field and emphasized that unless we control the frantic pace of the corporate treadmill, we may succumb from its pressures.

When his lab wasn't having subjects hold their arms in ice water to measure stress reactions, they were developing stress indexes. The following index was developed by Dr. Eliot at his Institute of Stress Medicine.

THE STRUGGLE INDEX*

Daily life can be a struggle. How do you deal with it? Do you talk to yourself? We all do. This is called self-talk. Negative self-talk can be harmful and self-defeating. But positive self-talk is a powerful way to bring about healthy change.

Let's measure your self-talk. How many of these items match your feelings? Indicate how strongly you agree with each of the following statements:

4 = all the time
3 = often
2 = sometimes
1 = never

_____ I am regularly exhausted by daily demands at work and home.

_____ My stress is caused by outside forces beyond my control.

_____ I am trapped by circumstances that I just have to live with.

_____ No matter how hard I work to stay on top of my schedule, I never feel caught up.

_____ I have financial obligations that I cannot meet.

_____ I dislike my work but cannot take the risk of a career change.

_____ I'm dissatisfied with my personal relationships.

_____ I feel responsible for the happiness of people around me.

_____ I am embarrassed to ask for help.

_____ I do not know what I want out of life.

_____ I am disappointed that I have not achieved what I had hoped for.

_____ No matter how much external success I have, I feel empty inside.

(continued on following page)

* "The Struggle Index," p. 164 in *From Stress to Strength: How to Lighten Your Load and Save Your Life*, Robert S. Eliot, M.D. (Published by Bantam Doubleday Dell, ©1994 Robert S. Eliot, M.D. Rights owned by Mrs. Phyllis Eliot. Reprinted with permission.)

_____ If the people around me were more competent, I would be happier.

_____ Many people have let me down in the past.

_____ I "stew" in my anger rather than express it.

_____ I become enraged and resentful when I am hurt.

_____ I can't take criticism.

_____ I am afraid I'll lose my job (home, finances, etc.)

_____ I do not see the value of expressing sadness or grief.

_____ I do not trust that things will work out.

_____ Total number of points

SCORING:

80–70 Life has become one crisis and struggle after another.

69–50 Your options are often clouded, and you feel trapped.

49–30 You have an awareness that your life is in your hands.

29–20 You are your own best ally with a high degree of control, self-esteem and identity.

You can buffer some of the slings and arrows that assault you every day. Because you are the author of your life, you can change the script and handle the stress of life more effectively.

- **Find joy in life.** Develop a genuine commitment for something that gives you great pleasure. Keep your passion going, whether it's coaching your child's soccer team, rummaging around old bookstores or collecting butterflies. Find time for relaxation. Clear your mind. Start with small chunks of time for yourself. Find things you enjoy outside of work and other obligations—paint, dance, take a course at a community college, for example.

- **Face challenges.** View difficulties as challenges to confront and master rather than as situations to flee from. Learn to see life as a challenge and opportunity even in your darkest moments. Most of us get frustrated with mistakes and failure when things don't work. Expect things not to work. When something fails, you might even think: *See, I told you, it wouldn't work.* Anticipate outcomes and ask yourself up front: What if it doesn't work? Don't let your decisions weigh you down like a rock around your neck. Figure out what you learned from the experience and move on.

- **Control what you can.** Focus on what you do have control over, not what you don't. When life is speeding along at two hundred miles per hour and seems out of control, what can you do to put the brakes on? Create boundaries between home and work or between other obligations such as caregiving. When home becomes work and work becomes home, physically separate your work space, for example. Close the mental—if not physical—door. Set times when you cannot be interrupted by family duties and vice versa.

- **Laugh.** The antidote to stress may just be laughter. If you're looking forward to a favorite comedy on TV, just checking the TV listings may trigger healthy mood changes, reduce your stress hormone levels and boost your immune system's defenses. A study presented at a Society for Neuroscience meeting was the first to show that anticipation of a mirthful event may be good for you. Lee Berk, assistant professor of family medicine, and his colleagues at the Susan Samueli Center for Complementary and Alternative Medicine at the University of California-Irvine, found that anticipating a laugh-inducing event reduced levels of tension, anger, depression, fatigue and confusion up to two days before the actual event. "We've demonstrated that watching a funny video can stimulate the body's ability to manage stress and fight disease," Dr. Berk said, referring to his previous research on the mood-enhancing effects of comedy. "But this is the first time we've seen that just anticipating such an event can change the body's responses. We believe this 'biology of hope' underlies recovery from many chronic disorders. Treatments that take advantage of the effects of this hope may go a long way to stimulating immune responses and hasten recovery."

Get a Life—Connectedness Can Happen

Study after study has documented that a sense of community, a sense of connectedness and a life partner to whom we can cling in times of stress may be measurable and workable solutions to finding sanity in the midst of chaos.

Here's how.

You've told your teenagers to "get a life" a million times when they sleep until noon and leave their dirty laundry around as if it will magically turn into folded, clean stacks. They act as if the world revolves around them. We're all teenagers in the sense that we all want the world to revolve around us, but what really works wellness-wise is getting out into the world and getting connected.

Connectedness can happen; we all want to be connected, to widen our social circle throughout life, not just at a time of crisis or illness. Let me offer some tried-and-true ways to do that:

- **Volunteer.** Studies have shown that older people who stay connected to others by volunteering live longer than those who don't volunteer. Certainly, your local hospital can use your help but so can schools. Read with elementary students. Tutor at a nearby high school. Visit someone who's caring for an ailing relative or friend. Serve lasagna at a homeless shelter. Offer your services to organizations that help victims of domestic violence. Deliver meals to the elderly. Become a foster family for your animal shelter. Work at the food bank. Give blood.

- **Share your knowledge.** Are you retired from law or business or sales? Hook up with organizations that assist new and small businesses. Teach gardening at the community college or offer personal enrichment programs such as quilting or picture framing through your school district. If photography is your hobby, teach it. If you always loved coaching your kids (or never made time) and now they're grown, coach other people's kids.

- **Work at your hobby.** Go ahead and buy the '64 Chevy Super Sport and restore it in your garage. Set a goal and make it happen. Browse a craft fair and engage an avid crafter to find out how you can get started making candles, stringing beaded bracelets or designing holiday ornaments. If you use your analytical left brain in your business and work life, maybe it's time to tap into the creative right side for better life balance.

- **Go back to school.** Learning is a lifelong activity. Take a class. Finish a degree. Earn college credit. Check out adult ed classes near you. Cooking and restaurant meal-tasting are popular, as are day trips to art museums and nearby historic sites.

- **Get a pet.** If you choose a dog, you'll have a ready-made walking partner. But pets can work magic in other ways, too: Teach your pet. Take your dog to obedience class. Or simply take your dog to the park, and enjoy Fido's ability to attract people.

- **Be a sport.** Attend local sporting events such as college basketball, youth soccer at the YMCA, league hockey, peewee baseball. Ask if you can help. And by all means join a wellness center where you can exercise your mind, body and spirit with others. Take the yoga class you always said you wanted to try.

- **Join something.** What interests you? Mystery writing? Duplicate bridge? Small engines? Cooking? Drumming? Tarot cards? Find a special interest group by scanning community calendars and online bulletin boards in your city, or create your own group by posting notices online or in the grocery store. Meet regularly at a local bookstore or coffee shop.

- **Attend worship services.** Studies show that older people who attend religious services live longer than those who don't attend services. Church groups are always seeking volunteers and making social events out of raking leaves, painting houses for the disadvantaged or conducting clothing drives.

Finding solace in a whisky bottle isn't on this list. Yet there is emerging evidence that alcohol clearly has beneficial medicinal value. Consistent studies document that a glass of red wine a day does exert some protective cardiovascular benefit against heart disease. On the other hand, we need to recognize the social devastation that can occur from inappropriate alcohol use, which I discuss in my next chapter.

My Thoughts . . .

One of the most important lessons in stress management is discovery of a sacred space where we can put on our emotional armor before heading back into the arena. This may be a stunning hiking trail in Glacier National Forest, a sweet fishing spot in the wilds of Northern Minnesota's Boundary Waters or a sugar-sand beach lapped by warm turquoise water. Your escape may be virtual—a mental vacation using imagery to take you to your sacred place when you can't physically go there.

We need to take a lesson from some of the world's great religious leaders. They took time to get away—to the mountains, to the desert—to become refreshed and renewed. Solitude is one of the keys to the kingdom.

Feeling too busy to take care of yourself? Not enough time to worry about diet and exercise or regular checkups? You'll have lots of time in the intensive-care unit when your heart decides to give you a wake-up call. Think about it. If you don't have time to get gas for your car, you'll pay later for sure when you're the one at the side of the road with the hood up. Same with your body.

6

Lifestyle: Choice Not Chance

As you walk down the fairway of life, you must smell the roses, for you only get to play one round.

—Ben Hogan

The handwriting is on the wall. Lifestyle choices do make a difference in how well we live and how long we live. In other words, we can prevent the vast majority of medical miseries, including cancer and heart disease, at least in part, by taking charge of our lives; by being proactive; by being an active participant in health-care decisions; and by recognizing that the buck stops with us when it comes to lifestyle choices such as drinking, smoking, sleeping and exposure to the sun.

I'll give you some practical, painless advice for quitting, moderating and improving in all of these areas.

Alcohol: Use Not Abuse

Some people should not drink alcohol. I'm one of them. After descending from four generations of alcoholics, I don't need to be told twice that alcohol and I simply won't mix. Others may enjoy a glass of red wine (just one) to avoid heart disease. But where alcohol use may spill over into abuse, moderation is the watchword. (In addition, alcohol can be harmful to many health conditions.)

Most studies seem to suggest that at least 10 percent of the American population is chemically dependent. No one can calculate alcohol's full role in marital discord, fatal automobile accidents, and/or the ruin of productive and creative lives. If you or someone you love is concerned about alcoholism, this clearly requires the input of a credentialed professional.

Many of us in clinical medicine use the phrase "CAGE" to assess when use becomes abuse. Now what does this mean?

C: Does anyone on a *consistent* basis complain about your drinking?

A: Do you become *annoyed* when someone comments about your drinking?

G: Are you drinking *greater* quantities of alcohol?

E: Do you require an *"eye opener"* to start the day, or are you drinking in the morning?

If an individual says yes to two or more of these four questions, we doctors raise a red flag about chemical dependency. The implications are far-reaching. A hallmark of alcoholism is denial, and it is very difficult for the individual to be objective about his or her own drinking habits. That is why we doctors need the input of family and community to help us determine the extent of the individual's chemical dependency.

A Mayo Clinic study in the journal *Cancer* looked at the interaction of alcohol and family history of breast cancer. Among women who had breast cancer, first-degree relatives (mother, sister or daughter) who drank alcohol daily had an increased risk for also developing breast cancer. For second-degree relatives (nieces) the risk was still there but less. By comparison, there was no increased risk for breast cancer among women who were related by marriage and still reported daily use of alcohol.

Moderation may apply to alcohol use, but it does not apply to the next subject: smoking.

The No-Smoking Section

If smokers stopped smoking, there would be short-term savings in health-care costs because smokers are known to have more disease than nonsmokers. But eventually, nationwide *smoking cessation would lead to increased health-care costs* as people live longer and incur more health costs at advanced ages *(The New England Journal of Medicine,* 1997) . . . think about it.

Smoking may be a tempting solution to curb rising health-care costs, but I don't subscribe to it.

Cigarette smoking has been on the decline in the United States over the past half century, moving from a high of 45 percent in 1954 to 23.5 percent today, according to government tracking sources. That's 46.5 million adults (with 3,000 teens joining those ranks every day).

- More men than women smoke.
- American Indians/Alaska Natives have the highest smoking rates (40.8 percent); Hispanics (18.1 percent) and Asians/Pacific Islanders (15.1 percent) the lowest.
- Adults who had earned a GED equivalent of a high-school diploma have high smoking rates (44.4 percent); those with higher college and professional degrees the lowest (8.5 percent).
- Those ages 18 to 24 had the highest rates (27.9 percent); those older than age 65 the lowest (10.6 percent).

Even so, among all these smokers, 76 percent of them would like to quit. Most smokers know it's harmful to themselves and others. They know it causes lung cancer, heart disease and other ills. Two-thirds of smokers have tried to quit. So why don't they?

IF YOU COULD TALK TO THE CEO OF A MAJOR TOBACCO COMPANY, WHAT WOULD YOU ASK?

Brown & Williamson Tobacco Chairman and CEO Nick Brookes took questions from the public on an Internet chat. Here are a couple of his responses:

Q: **How do you account for your company's historic denial of the addictive and poisonous nature of nicotine?**

A: Our position . . . is that *smoking is addictive,* as that term is understood by most people today in America. However, I personally believe that it's not appropriate to use that term if the intention in doing so is to somehow lump our consumers together with heroin and crack-cocaine addicts, or indeed, to suggest that the hard-working tobacco farmers of Kentucky, North Carolina and Virginia are no better than the coca farmers of Colombia or the heroin poppy farmers of Cambodia. Such comparisons in my opinion are ludicrous. It can be tough to quit, but there is nothing in cigarettes to prevent smokers from reaching and implementing a decision to quit. Indeed, there are more people today who have smoked and quit than there are folks that continue to smoke. [In an earlier question, Brookes admitted that he had quit smoking eleven months earlier to support his wife who had quit smoking.]

Q: **Are you willing to go on record to acknowledge that the causative link between cigarettes and lung cancer has been conclusively proven?**

A: We accept that the best judgment on all the evidence is that *smoking causes lung cancer.*

Finally, more than thirty-five years after the U.S. Surgeon General Dr. Luther Terry released the first Surgeon General's report on smoking and health in 1964, the tobacco industry admitted blame. Dr. Terry's 387-page report on the link between smoking and cancer and other serious diseases was released on a Saturday because reports say that President Lyndon Johnson was concerned that its contents would have an effect on the stock market. This was the first official word from Washington on the cause-and-effect relationship between smoking and disease. Today, the official word is inscribed on every cigarette pack sold.

But even this knowledge has done little to make a difference. Lung cancer has reached epidemic proportions in this country and is a major killer of women, too. If tobacco-related cancers were eliminated, the war on cancer would certainly be a success.

Tobacco industry insider, Jeffrey Wigand, Ph.D., the whistle-blower whose story was told in the movie *The Insider,* tells audiences across the country that cigarettes are the only product that "when used as intended, kill you." He looks nothing like the actor Russell Crowe, by the way, who played his role so brilliantly for Hollywood, but Dr. Wigand doesn't need glitz and glamour to make his points:

- There is no "safe cigarette." But the tobacco industry is attempting to polish its image in the aftermath of the massive tobacco settlement by developing so-called safer products. The newer models may be lower in tar, but the extra baggage that comes along with the nicotine has four to eight times the amount of carbon monoxide than regular smokes. "If you want carbon monoxide," Dr. Wigand suggests, "go suck the exhaust of a school bus."

- Although cigarettes are unregulated and require no ingredients label like foods do, the list of ingredients would include 599 different chemicals intended to maintain their hold on addicted smokers. Some of these ingredients are so toxic and carcinogenic (cancer-causing), you cannot dispose of them legally in this country—except through cigarettes.

- To break the bonds of smoking's chemical and physical addiction, Dr. Wigand suggests nicotine-replacement therapy plus medication and behavioral modification. Even at that, only half of people will be able to quit. Smokers often try five times before they become successful quitters.

The vast majority of lung cancers are directly related to cigarette smoking, even though a small minority of patients who never smoked will get lung cancer. If the cancer cannot be surgically removed, only a small percentage of patients are alive at five years. The average survival for patients with advanced lung cancer is less than a year.

Bladder cancer is yet another disease linked to smoking. Cigarette smokers are two to three times more likely than nonsmokers to get bladder cancer—the fourth most common cancer in men and the eighth most common among women. Scientists at UCLA's Jonsson Cancer Center are looking into whether green tea extract and experimental drugs can act as preventive agents. Nothing prevents better than not smoking at all—or quitting if you do smoke.

Cigars—A safer alternative to cigarettes?

The allure of a fine cigar has shaped public perception and misinformation about them. The glamorous image of cigar smokers clouds the issue: The real issue is that cigar smoking, like cigarette smoking, is known to cause lung cancer. Rates of cigar smoking are rising among adults and adolescents (among both teenage boys and girls). Many see cigars as a safer alternative to cigarettes, but they are not.

Smoking cigars instead of cigarettes does not reduce the risk of nicotine addiction either. And the more you inhale, the more your risk of death related to cigar smoking increases—and may reach as high a risk level as that for smoking cigarettes.

Are cigars a safer alternative to cigarettes? No, say researchers in *The Journal of the American Medical Association*. The fundamental difference between cigars and cigarettes is the processing. And it's the curing and fermenting of tobacco for cigars to achieve the desired flavor and aroma that may increase a long list of nasty ingredients that eventually increase the amount of free nicotine in cigars.

Just a pinch

Use of smokeless tobacco, either as dip (tobacco placed between the lip and gum) or chew (chewed tobacco) has increased among young white men who think, incorrectly, that it's a healthier choice than smoking cigarettes. Its use is strongly linked to cancer of the mouth, vocal cords—and everything else down to the stomach. Two bits of news:

- Dental hygienists at the Oregon Research Institute talked about the mouth sores, bleeding and receding gums they observed among smokeless tobacco users who came for annual dental cleanings. Among these patients who were also given a self-help video, quit rates tripled compared with patients who received the usual care and no health education advice.

- Even better news comes from U.S. Air Force researchers. For patients who stopped using smokeless tobacco, potentially precancerous mouth sores healed completely within six weeks of quitting.

For some reason, the nicotine replacement products, such as patches and gum, haven't seemed to help smokeless tobacco users quit. But my colleagues in the Mayo Nicotine Research Center have done a small study with measurable success and some lessons. The study was published in the journal *Nicotine and Tobacco Research*.

They used the antidepressant bupropion (brand name Zyban or Wellbutrin) with a test group of spit tobacco users and compared that with a control group given a placebo (a pill with no active ingredients). Neither group, of course, knew if they were getting the active drug, which is the hallmark of sound research.

After twelve weeks, 44 percent of the active drug users had stopped tobacco use compared with 26 percent of those using no active drug. This does say that there is some usefulness in any study with a placebo, but the results are good news for smokeless tobacco users who feel they need some help quitting.

This is doubly good news because 12 to 16 percent of young men chew tobacco, I'm told. It's a significant enough problem that having a successful treatment option is important. Like street drugs, peer pressure to use smokeless tobacco can be a powerful factor. In fact, smokeless tobacco has been called a gateway "drug" for smoking. Men were found to be more than 2.5 times as likely to have switched from smokeless tobacco to cigarettes than to have substituted snuff for smokes. These observations were made in a very large national survey conducted by the CDC and published in the *American Journal of Preventive Medicine*.

Don't inhale

Marijuana use increases risk for head or neck cancers. Researchers from UCLA, publishing in the journal *Cancer Epidemiology*, found that subjects in their study who had used marijuana were more than twice as likely to develop these deadly cancers. The more marijuana the subjects used, the greater their risk. Marijuana smoke contains as much as 50 percent higher concentrations of known cancer-causing substances and deposits four times as much tar in the respiratory tract as one cigarette does.

I can't make a case for tobacco use at all in any form, but I can make some observations about ending this horrible habit no matter what form of nicotine you ingest.

Even hard-core smokers can quit

Imagine a research study of smokers who have smoked for an average of twenty-two years, most of whom have tried to quit in the past. They average more than a pack a day. Many have their first cigarette of the day within fifteen minutes of waking up (an indicator that they are dependent on tobacco). That was the challenge in a recent study using nicotine gum plus tailored health messages. Bottom line: The combination of nicotine replacement and education was twice as likely to work—and helped longtime smokers quit for good.

"When a person decides to quit smoking using nicotine replacement therapy [this study used nicotine gum and was sponsored by its manufacturer], having personalized self-help materials . . . significantly improves their success," said a researcher who directs the Smoking Research Group at the University of Pittsburgh.

Smokers were given individualized information by mail based on their goals for quitting, their smoking history, their lack of success in quitting in the past, their target quit date and the difficulties they expected. These tailored programs are often available through state smoking quitlines, through your employer and even from the pharmaceutical companies that make nicotine-replacement products. Use them.

So far thirty-three states have instituted phone-based quitlines, and so have large managed-care plans. In California alone, more than fifty-five thousand tobacco users call the quitlines each year for programs conducted in six languages.

It's hard for anyone to quit smoking, but women may have a tougher time, according to research reviewing several studies and published in the journal *CNS Drugs,* according to the National Institute of Drug Abuse. Researchers suggest that antidepressant medication used for smoking cessation (Zyban), rather than nicotine gum or patches, may be more effective for women than for men. Here's why:

- Women smokers are more fearful than men of gaining a lot of weight if they quit. The additional weight gain, if any, is far healthier than the damage the smoking is doing, even if smoking keeps off a few pounds.

- Husbands may provide less effective support to women who are trying to quit smoking than wives give to husbands.
- Women may be more susceptible than men to environmental cues to smoking, such as smoking with certain friends or smoking associated with specific moods.
- Many women may enjoy the feeling of control associated with smoking a cigarette.

Just as men are more apt to quit "cold turkey," women, because they are from a different planet, will stop and ask for directions. Therefore, women are more likely to ask for help when trying to quit smoking, according to a national Yankelovich survey conducted for the National Women's Health Resource Center. With so many quitting options for smokers, it's critical for smokers to enlist the support of their doctors.

But is your doctor prepared to help you quit?

We're not doing enough in our medical schools to train medical students to help their patients quit smoking. Part of the problem is that we simply don't know how to teach behavior change to our up-and-coming colleagues.

Some of the leading schools are using role-playing techniques with pretend patients, according to a report in *The Journal of the American Medical Association*. But most med schools still rely on traditional lectures and handouts, and students may have as few as three hours on smoking-cessation techniques—imagine, just three hours in a four-year program.

Here is the irony. Several studies have shown that smokers would quit if their doctor told them to. But when nicotine replacement therapies such as patches and gum became available over-the-counter and did not require a doctor's prescription, in mid-1996, their effectiveness in helping people quit went down. Why? Because doctors were not in the loop on the counseling end anymore. When a doctor prescribed the gum or patch, the doctor would discuss your need and the use of the product to curb cravings for nicotine. But when nicotine replacement products were available practically everywhere, smokers were not getting the behavioral counseling component so essential to quitting. Smokers' quitlines may help replace some of the professional counseling needed to boost the effectiveness of these products.

Doctors, however, can be your best ally when you tackle this lifelong addiction. Older smokers (sixty-five-plus years of age) are more likely to quit smoking or remain nonsmoking if they see a doctor and dentist on a regular basis, according to Canadian research in the *Journal of Gerontology: Medical Sciences.* Just having a regular physician and seeing a dentist regularly was a remarkable predictor of who smoked and who didn't. Smokers in the study of over seventy-three thousand people were much less likely to have seen a dentist in the past five years and didn't have a regular doctor.

In the early days of Hollywood, the movies portrayed smoking seductively: the couple enjoying a romantic, smoke-filled moment. Today, some couples who smoke together find it extremely difficult to break that bond, despite overwhelming evidence that smoking kills. An antismoking campaign in Oregon uses a Hollywood scene to encourage quitting: He says, "Mind if I smoke?" and she replies, "Care if I die?"

Many couples, after smoking for years together, find that smoking is an integral part of their relationship, according to Michael Rohrbaugh, professor of family studies and human development and psychology, University of Arizona. When one person seeks to quit, the dynamics of the relationship can change. His research shows that family and relationship patterns contribute to continuing high-risk smoking.

The ongoing challenge for research is to develop treatment programs for single-smoker couples and what to do for couples who smoke when one quits.

Are you prepared to help yourself? Here are a few techniques:

- **Declare a smokefree home,** and your chances of quitting smoking are higher. Smokefree homes give family members an effective means of exerting social pressure on smokers living with them and a powerful tool for changing the smokers' behavior, say scientists at the Cancer Prevention and Control Program at the University of California-San Diego.

- **Fight or switch?** At one time, smokers would rather fight than switch brands. But now, smokers who switch are more likely to be quitters. If smokers switch to lower-tar or -nicotine cigarettes for health reasons, they are more likely to quit smoking compared with those who smoke regular cigarette brands, according to researchers in the *Annals of Behavioral Medicine.* Switchers in the study of thousands of Air Force recruits, who were hoping to reduce their health risks, were less dependent on nicotine and were more likely to have tried to quit smoking before. They also made better lifestyle choices by choosing higher intakes of fruits and vegetables, less high-fat food, and were less likely to drive fast and more likely to use safety belts.

- **Never quit quitting.** Often, people relapse if they smoke one cigarette or an entire pack while they're trying to quit. If this happens to you, you have not failed. The best thing to do is to try to quit again *as soon as possible.* After so much mental and physical preparation, such as choosing a quit date and talking with your doctor about medications that may ease the transition, it's much easier to try again soon after a relapse than to try to quit several weeks or months later. Don't put too much pressure on yourself. The first few days after you quit, you may temporarily feel tired, irritable, and develop headaches or a cough. Keep in mind you're taking the first step toward better health—even though it may not seem so at the time. Never quit quitting until you really do.

Smoking doesn't affect me; I don't smoke

Think again.

When dining out, you certainly want to be comfortable and enjoy your meal. You don't want dinner spoiled by toxic chemicals floating in the air. So the last place you'd choose to eat is next to a busy highway or waste dump, right? Yet that's exactly what happens when someone lights a cigarette in a restaurant, according to the Environmental Protection Agency.

Restaurants that allow smoking can have six times the pollution of a busy highway. Secondhand smoke has many of the same poisons as the air around a toxic waste dump, says the American Cancer Society.

Don't be fooled. Restaurants that have separate smoking and nonsmoking sections cannot eliminate your exposure to the toxins from secondhand smoke. Ventilation systems are designed to efficiently circulate air within the enclosed environment, not to filter and clean it. Trying to have a smokefree section of a restaurant is like trying to have a chlorine-free section of a swimming pool.

If you must eat in a restaurant that is not entirely smokefree, I suggest you ask to be seated as far as possible from where people are smoking. Contrary to fears that restaurants would lose business by going smokefree, in cities where ordinances prohibit smoking entirely in restaurants, business is booming. More than 75 percent of adult Americans do not smoke (and they like to dine out).

Protect your children from exposure to secondhand smoke, too. More than 40 percent of children in the United States live in homes where at least one adult smokes. Being exposed increases a child's risk for developing asthma or worsening existing asthma, according to the American Academy of Allergy, Asthma, and Immunology. This group, along with the Environmental Protection Agency and other national organizations, encourages parents who smoke to do so outside their homes. This goes for guests in your home and for babysitters, and should be something you consider when looking at day-care centers.

Tobacco smoke is more harmful to children than to adults because their lungs still are developing. Researchers at Massachusetts General Hospital addressed parents' smoking habits when their children were admitted to the hospital for respiratory illnesses. The thinking is that the illness was caused or made worse by exposure to secondhand smoke. Many parents who were targeted in this "teachable moment" took advantage of smoking cessation programs the hospital offered.

Like canaries in mine shafts, children can show the harm from passive smoking first. But for adults, by the time symptoms of lung cancer evolve, such as a nasty cough, pain or bloody sputum, most patients are beyond cure. When diagnosed with lung cancer, many smokers express regret at having smoked. But feeling guilty at that point is not constructive and wastes energy. Even with advanced cancer, it's time to stop smoking because patients who stop smoking may be more fit and better able to tolerate therapy.

Major advances have been made in the treatment of this disaster, but, generally, the final victory is not really in sight. Routine chest x-rays are not a helpful tool in diagnosis, but there is some exciting news. The spiral CT scans detect cancers when they are far smaller than with a chest x-ray. The high-risk person may want to check into this screening method, but it has not yet been recommended as a screening tool for whole populations.

If you cannot stop smoking, decrease the number of cigarettes you smoke. In one year, fewer than 3 percent of smokers quit by themselves. This is not a moral flaw. It's difficult. But talk with your doctor. Patches, medications, gum, inhalers, lozenges and support—sometimes in combination with each other—are working. The time is right, the best time is now. No doubt, smoking is the most preventable cause of death and disease.

Sleep: Not Enough Zzzzzzzs

You're heard the word *circadian* used to describe sleep cycles. Circadian is a rhythm associated with our twenty-four-hour sleep/wake cycle, and it is set by the twenty-four-hour trip our earth takes to rotate once around its axis from day to night and back again. For most of us, these rotations become regular and downright routine. But if something disrupts that routine—like jet travel to Europe or shiftwork on the job—you can throw off your entire metabolism, including sleep.

The body's circadian clock is a tiny cluster of nerve cells behind your eyes. These cells send out the signals that control your natural daily rhythms.

We are a sleep-deprived society. Our generation gets less sleep than almost any other in American history. Overall, Americans are getting at least 20 percent less sleep than they did one hundred years ago (TV and the Internet are causing almost half of adults to stay up later than they should), and our 24/7 society is seeing a dramatic drop in productivity because of it.

Results from a poll on Sleep in America, taken by the National Sleep Foundation (NSF), may be a wake-up call. Sleep loss takes a toll. Look at what lack of sleep is doing to the American workplace:

- 51 percent of working Americans say sleepiness on the job interferes with the amount of work they get done.
- 49 percent admit the quality of their work suffers when they are sleepy.
- 27 percent say they are sleepy at work two or more days a week.
- 24 percent have difficulty getting up for work two or more days per week.
- 19 percent report making occasional or frequent work errors because of sleepiness.

The NSF estimates the direct cost to employers at $18 billion (in 1997) for decreased productivity, work errors and absenteeism. One solution: Napping on the job (a third of adults interviewed said they would nap at work if allowed). This is a logical solution unless, of course, you drive a truck or work in a nuclear plant for a living.

Sleep deprivation may explain why accidents happen. There is no doubt that insomnia is a national epidemic clearly affecting worker safety and worker productivity. The errors that lead up to many catastrophes occur in the early hours of the morning when someone's attention span is clearly limited and when fatigue was probably an overriding factor.

A number of Mediterranean and Latin American countries have instituted the concept of the midday siesta. From a biological and from a physiological standpoint, this makes perfectly good sense, especially during the heat of the day. However, as the world becomes increasingly digitalized and Westernized, this practice is becoming eroded, much to the detriment of body and soul.

Asleep at the wheel

Driving without proper rest can be as risky as driving drunk. Sleepy drivers are much more likely to be involved in a sleep-related crash, says the American Automobile Association Foundation for Traffic Safety and research from the North Carolina Highway Safety Research Center.

A sleepy driver may be your neighbor who is putting in extra hours at work or a new parent sleep-deprived because Baby keeps night hours. Often, overly tired drivers report not knowing how sleepy they really are and say they don't feel sleepy before driving.

The typical drowsy driver is more likely to

- work night shifts
- work sixty or more hours a week
- work more than one job
- take medications that may cause drowsiness
- sleep less than six hours per night, leading to sleep deprivation
- be awake for twenty hours or longer
- drive frequently between midnight and 6:00 A.M.

It all adds up to risk of falling asleep behind the wheel and the potential for a serious crash. Let this be a wake-up call to every driver to pay attention to sleeping patterns and plan not to drive while sleep-deprived. The old methods of turning up the radio or opening a window simply do not keep drowsy drivers awake. Only sleep can.

Losing sleep in your quest for rest?

Various sleep disorders can affect whether you have a good night's sleep. The composer of one of the world's best-known lullabies (hum along with me: "lullaby and good night") may have suffered from a common sleep disorder known as sleep apnea. Researchers have speculated that Johannes Brahms (1833–1897) had sleep apnea, which affects as many as 20 million Americans. Doctors in his day, however, were unaware of the risks of the condition.

Sleep apnea causes a sudden interruption of breathing, heavy snoring, sleep deprivation and excessive daytime sleepiness. Brahms never married, but a traveling companion said no one could sleep in the same room because of his snoring. The rather large Brahms (obesity is another risk factor for sleep apnea) was known to snooze in the afternoon in the Vienna cafes—he was a familiar sight for gawking tourists.

Fortunately, new techniques are helping many with sleep apnea get relief and a sound sleep (and their bed partners, too). With proper medical help for sleep apnea, no one would need a lullaby—not even dear old Johannes Brahms.

Bright news about the dark days of winter

With the October end of daylight savings time in most parts of the country, millions of Americans may be plunged into the darkness of shorter winter days with a condition called seasonal affective disorder (also known as SAD).

Our internal body clocks—the circadian clock—depend on light signals to tell us when to be energetic and when to sleep. That's why we tend to be more active in summer and less productive in winter. There really may be something to hibernation after all!

Getting out of bed on a dark winter morning can be tough. It's especially hard in Rochester, Minnesota. I've survived over thirty winters here, so I know. But for millions of people with seasonal affective disorder, it's even worse. Their body clocks need a strong stimulus of light, like sunlight, to reset their circadian rhythms every day. In winter, they don't receive this strong light signal, so their internal body clock shifts and produces the wrong hormones at the wrong time of day.

As the season wears on, this imbalance can cause fatigue, exhaustion and even depression. People with SAD may have trouble sleeping, can be unable to concentrate, and lack energy and alertness.

Talk with your doctor about symptoms of SAD. Light treatment is often recommended, in which people sit in front of full-spectrum light to reset that internal clock. Other strategies can often help:

- Try to keep a consistent sleep/wake cycle.
- Increase the overall light in your home, especially in the morning and evening, and stay in well-lit areas.
- Make sure evening activities include light. Don't watch TV, for example, in the dark.
- Be active! Physical activities decrease the effects of shifted circadian rhythms.

There is a school of thought among Eastern healers that the time you wake up, if you wake up in the night, tells you what's troubling you. So, for example, if you awaken prematurely between midnight and 2:00 A.M., you're feeling anger, so they say. Waking between 2:00 and 4:00 A.M. signifies fear, and if you're up watching infomercials from 4:00 to 6:00 A.M., you're feeling sadness.

I don't know how much truth there is to this theory, but lack of sleep for any reason—sleep apnea, shiftwork, depression, seasonal affective disorder, a snoring bed partner—is reason enough to talk with your doctor about what may be causing it.

Back Pain: The Lowdown

With back pain, sometimes the best medicine is no medicine (or surgery) at all.

Disability claims and medical expenses for back-related injuries and illnesses approach hundreds of millions of dollars a year. For the vast majority of people with back pain and injury, surgery is not the answer because most people will get better with conservative management that includes rest, heat, massage and anti-inflammatory medications—and time. The medications used include ibuprofen and other over-the-counter medications known as nonsteroidal anti-inflammatories (NSAIDs). Brand names include Motrin and Aleve.

You can avoid many back-pain-related injuries by using the following tips:

- Use your hands and knees when lifting heavy objects. A fifty-pound weight held at arm's length will generate twelve hundred pounds of pressure on the lower part of your back. Hold heavy items close to your body or don't lift them at all without help.
- Listen to your body. Most people have a premonition of back tightness or spasm. Be wise—don't ignore that little voice. Always be cautious about lifting objects and never try to be a hero.
- Within reason, avoid repetitive activities. Persistent heavy lifting, gardening, outdoor work and golf can put a tremendous strain on your lower spine. Warm up, and don't think you need to prove you're macho. Remember, you are not nineteen years old anymore.
- Recognize your limitations. As a general rule of thumb, if you are more than age forty or fifty, you should not lift more than thirty to forty pounds.

No Safe Sun: Indoors or Out

One morning, I walked into the exam room where a young mother was breastfeeding her newborn. Beside her were her husband and her parents. She had been diagnosed with malignant melanoma (black-mole cancer, the deadliest form of skin cancer). She was dying. Her life was in my hands—as have been the lives of over fifty-five thousand patients I have seen in my thirty-year career as a cancer specialist.

Later the same day, another young woman was awaiting me in a hospital bed. She too had malignant melanoma that began as a freckle on her left thigh. Because her situation was so grave, she had moved up her wedding date. She was to be married in ten days because a planned summer wedding, just three months away, seemed far too long to wait. As I was leaving her bedside, she held out her hand and embraced mine. "Please pray with me," she said. I did.

The young mother's cancer began with an itchy mole on her neck. Both women had tanned as teenagers so they could look bronzed in their prom dresses. They didn't expect those strapless gowns to be part of a chain of events that would lead to their horrible diagnoses and to me.

Here's the issue: *malignant melanoma*. This is one of the most deadly forms of cancer that we oncologists see. It is increasing faster than any other cancer, even faster than lung cancer and breast cancer. The real tragedy and the real opportunity is that malignant melanoma is completely preventable. This is a cancer caused, in large measure, by exposure to the sun.

We've all heard the message, but is anyone listening?

The American Academy of Dermatology—representing the skin doctors who first see the harmful and sometimes fatal effects of too much sun—is alarmed by the number of teenagers and young adults who continue to tan indoors and out and with the number of Americans who still think there is "safe sun."

There is no such thing as a safe tan. Think about what tanning means. When you expose your skin to the sun, ultraviolet radiation causes a reaction in the melanocytes (these are the skin cells that produce pigment or color), and your skin turns brown (theoretically, unless you've sunburned, which is even worse). The problem is not the brown color but the ultraviolet radiation that triggers a response in your DNA. Cells may go haywire and form a melanoma or other types of skin cancer.

The sunless tanners or "tan in a bottle" products can turn your skin brown or give it a bronze glow. These products put a nontoxic, simple sugar called DHA on your skin. Proteins in your skin interact with the sugars to create a tan. Though harmless, these products perpetuate the myth that a tan is good. A tan is not good. Somehow we need to change the attitude that people look better with a tan. They don't. They look like skin cancer waiting to happen.

Consider this: We use the process of tanning to turn animal skins into leather. When you process your skin under the sun, you allow the ultraviolet radiation to break down the proteins in your skin cells. Over time, you end up with premature aging and wrinkled leathery skin. It's your "hide."

Those seemingly simple sunburns that happen to teens and younger kids on beaches and at swimming pools and lakes across the country can be tracked to serious skin cancers later in life. More than half of teenagers report being sunburned within the past year, in a study published in the *American Journal of Preventive Medicine*. People who say, "I burn first, then I tan," are putting themselves at great risk. Interestingly, people in the states of Colorado, Iowa, Michigan, Indiana, Wyoming, Utah and Wisconsin, and in the District of Columbia, were more likely to sunburn than people in states such as Florida and Arizona where the sun shines for outdoor activities nearly all year. Perhaps these Sun Belt residents are getting the message.

Still, dermatologists are treating more and more fatal skin cancers in remarkably young patients. The common denominator is overexposure to the sun before the age of eighteen when their skin cells are especially vulnerable to injury from the sun's rays.

More than a million people a day invest time and money (and put their health at risk) in tanning salons. The damage they receive from indoor lamps is just as dangerous as outdoor sun exposure. Most salon bulbs provide a significant amount of UVA and UVB radiation—and both types of ultraviolet radiation are also found in the outdoor sun and can cause various types of damage.

"If you think you look better with a little sun, even though you are aware of the health risks of overexposure to the sun or think wearing sunscreen helps you prevent sunburn and get a good base tan, you're not alone," according to Mark Naylor, M.D., associate professor at the University of Oklahoma Health Science Center, reporting on a recent survey by the American Academy of Dermatology.

Most people surveyed knew that too much exposure to the sun is unhealthy, but 81 percent still think they look good after having been out in the sun. "A tan is still considered a standard of beauty, and people may believe that avoiding a sunburn by use of sunscreens makes tanning a safe activity and it doesn't," said Dr. Naylor.

"Using a sunscreen is popular because it is an easy way to practice sun safety without making a major change in your behavior," Dr. Naylor said. "Sunscreen should be used to reduce exposure to the sun and prevent premature aging and skin cancer, not to aid in getting a tan. Using a sunscreen to increase sun exposure during intentional tanning tends to defeat its purpose."

Think of your skin as being eight minutes away from the sun. Damaging ultraviolet rays travel the 93 million miles in eight minutes to inflict their harm. Stop the rays, choose your cover, and you'll lower your lifetime risk for skin cancer. You may even prevent other problems the sun causes to unprotected skin, and I'm talking about wrinkles—a sign not only of aging but of skin damage.

THE RULES TO PREVENT
SKIN CANCER FROM SUN EXPOSURE

- Use plenty (a generous handful for your entire body) of broad-spectrum sunscreen with SPF 15 or higher and reapply every two hours you are out in the sun. Studies show that most people apply much less sunscreen than is required to achieve the SPF (sun protection factor). More is better, in this case. If you apply less, then consider that you may not get the full SPF protection.

- Apply sunscreen to dry skin thirty minutes before being in the sun so it can be absorbed by the skin and is less likely to wash off when you perspire. Note expiration dates because some sunscreen ingredients can degrade over time.

- Don't wait until your skin begins to turn red to apply sunscreen. The damage has already begun.

- There are seventeen active ingredients approved for use in the United States. Sunscreens with inorganic ingredients such as titanium dioxide and zinc oxide reflect and scatter the damaging ultraviolet rays. Other organic ingredients such as OMC or avobenzone absorb and scatter the ultraviolet light as heat. A combination of these ingredients is often called broad-spectrum and helps get SPF factors higher. The higher the number, the more protection against sunburn, but that doesn't mean you should stay out longer in the sun. When buying your next sunscreen, read the labels just as carefully as you read food labels.

- Wear hats and protective clothing.

- Avoid outdoor activities when the sun's rays are the strongest: Follow the Shadow Rule: If your shadow is shorter than you are, the sun's damaging rays are at their strongest, and you are likely to sunburn.

- Seek shade but don't depend on it. Researchers at Purdue University created models showing the benefits of tree cover. They caution that even a tight canopy of leaves and branches cannot completely block the sun's rays and does not fully protect you from harmful sun. So much for that hammock!

As the most common form of cancer in the United States, skin cancer will be diagnosed more than a million times this year, and one person dies of its most fatal form, melanoma, every hour.

Let's talk about the signs and symptoms that might suggest a malignant melanoma:

- Unlike other cancers, you can see skin cancer. It appears on the surface of the skin. Pay attention to spots that appear and then go away, only to come back in the same place. Watch for areas that are easily irritated when you towel-dry yourself. These are tiny warning signs, so listen to them. Schedule a monthly self-exam.

- A mole or freckle that bleeds, itches, or changes color or texture needs to be seen by a physician. Every doctor's visit is an opportunity for a skin check—even when you're there for something else. So ask your doctor to take a look, especially in areas you cannot see easily, such as your back, back of your neck and scalp. You must take the initiative because primary care doctors only conduct skin exams at about 16 percent of office visits and talk to their patients about skin cancer prevention at just 2 percent of their visits, according to a study in the *Journal of General Internal Medicine*.

- A new mole or freckle, whether it is colored or not, should be evaluated by a physician. Pay attention to a mole that changes in color, shape or size. One study in the *Archives of Dermatology* noted that patients often don't realize a mole is changing or enlarging. If you're concerned about a spot, I suppose you could attempt to measure it. Better yet, get it looked at and spare yourself the uncertainty.

- Ask your spouse or partner to look at your back, and if there is an irregular or darkly pigmented spot, don't ignore it. Melanoma and other skin cancers can show up in areas that have never been exposed to the sun, so don't overlook any body area, including between your toes, in your scalp and on your genitals. More than half of people with melanomas found their own cancers. Women were more likely to detect theirs than men, and wives were more likely to spot something on their husbands than vice versa, according to a study by researchers at Memorial Sloan-Kettering Cancer Center reported in the journal *Cancer*. Physicians, however, did a good job of finding early skin cancer, especially if the patient had a family history of melanoma. Family history is important information you need to know and tell your doctors.

- A quick phone call to your local American Cancer Society can provide some very easy-to-use pamphlets that give more information on this deadly problem. And check the self-care sites on the Internet (recommended sites are listed at the end of this book) for illustrations and explanations as well.

Par for the course

You don't have to be a beach-dwelling sunbather to have reason for concern. I'm in just as much danger because, I will admit it, I am a golf addict. My exposure to the game (and the sun) started as a small boy in New Jersey as a caddy for some of the "very rich and very famous." The exclusive country club was right outside New York City, and I had the opportunity to caddy for captains of industry, celebrities, athletes and politicians.

Golf is enjoying an unprecedented boom. Currently, approximately 30 million Americans play golf. My guess is that you either play golf or know someone who enjoys this challenging game. In addition, 41 million more individuals are highly interested in golf or expect to play in the future, according to a marketing survey.

Golf obviously is an outdoor activity, and golfers need to be as crystal clear on the risks of melanoma as they need to be crystal clear on the risks of lightning.

Yet golfers who know the par on every hole and the score they had three summers ago are still relatively clueless about the dangers of the sun. A National Golf Foundation survey indicated that only 20 percent of golfers always use sunblock. To be on a golf course and not use sunscreen is the equivalent of sitting on the railroad tracks. Sooner or later you're going to get run over, and the results will not be pretty.

So what do we need to know? We need to know the SPF (sun protection factor) in sunscreen. The magic number is fifteen (15). Buy and use sunscreen that blocks both ultraviolet A and ultraviolet B radiation. This is clearly marked on the new labels that spell out the Sun Alert information. Forget about "all-day protection" and "waterproof." They're not.

Liberally apply the sunblock before playing golf, or going outside for any activity, and reapply every several holes, especially if you are actively perspiring. Most people don't apply enough. Rub on a good ounce, not just a dab here and there in vulnerable spots. In this case, more is better.

Some other tips are really important:

- Wear a broad-brimmed hat, much like Tom Kite or Greg Norman. The traditional golf cap or baseball cap does not shield the face and neck from the risks of the sun.
- Wear three-quarter-length sleeves. Make every reasonable effort to decrease sun exposure. If it were an ideal world, one would not tee off between 11:00 A.M. and 1:00 P.M., but, unfortunately, life is not fair, good tee times fill up fast, and we have to plan our schedules according to our work and our partners' schedules.
- Shorts are fine, but don't forget the sun exposure on the thighs and calves.

Golf is a great game. Let's live long enough to have at least one hole in one (let me tell you about mine!).

Winter sun: It's good for you

It's one of life's cruel ironies, but for most people, some sun is one of the best sources of vitamin D. This important nutrient makes your bones stronger and helps prevent fractures. You need about twenty minutes of sun each day, on the areas of your body that are normally exposed (such as your face and hands), to cause the chemical reaction in your skin that produces vitamin D.

How to get the sun you need: Sunlight that comes through window glass won't cause your skin to make vitamin D. But even in the winter, you don't have to park yourself in a lawn chair in the snow to get your twenty minutes of direct sunshine. In fact, you don't need to get it all at one time. You can add up the minutes of exposure you get from activities such as walking to the end of your driveway, to the bus stop or through the shopping mall parking lot to your car.

Vitamin D can be found supplemented in milk and in other foods. If you take a calcium supplement, make sure you're getting vitamin D either in the calcium pills themselves or separately through sun or food.

But if you can't get direct sunlight and decide to take vitamin D in pill form, ask your doctor for guidance first. It would be virtually impossible to overdose on vitamin D from sun exposure, but vitamin D supplements have harmful side effects if you take too much.

My Thoughts . . .

We are creatures of habit. We thrive on habit (good ones) and the routine of life. Results from research conducted on thousands of people over three decades show clear secrets to living a longer, healthier life. And I have embellished on this research from my colleague Lester Breslow, M.D., to give you some practical suggestions.

The secret to living a long and healthy life is not to be found in a tabloid headline, in a pill or potion, or in a diet plan. The secret is found within yourself and in what you do (and don't do) every day, day after day. Dr. Breslow and his colleagues consistently found these health habits to be the ones to follow:

1. Don't smoke. If you do, stop now.
2. Drink moderately or don't drink at all.
3. Get a good night's sleep of seven or eight hours.
4. Get up off the couch and get moving in some regular fashion thirty minutes at a time, several times a week. Walking vigorously is a top choice.
5. Forget the scales. Eat moderately so you maintain your weight in relation to your height.
6. Eat regularly, whether that's two meals a day, three, or five. Whatever you normally do, keep it up. It's the regularity of life and moderation in your eating, sleeping and exercising that makes all the difference.
7. Eat breakfast every day for sure.

To these magic seven, I add social connectedness. I see the value of social support, in having family and friends and activities you love as part of health and healing.

We Americans are now living longer than ever in history. The average individual life span at the turn of the twentieth century was the late forties. A high proportion of the population can now expect to live to at least eighty years of age and possibly far longer if these prudent guidelines are followed. The choice is up to each of us to make those years productive, creative and meaningful, as opposed to years of decrepitude dealing with the ravages not only of age but also of severe chronic illnesses.

The choice is always there. The information is available to help guide us in appropriate directions. Cancer or heart disease or diabetes or whatever is lurking in your family tree is not a "done deal," nor is it a case of roulette, a random selection of cards or a roll of the dice. We can put ourselves behind the eight-ball, deal ourselves a lousy hand, give ourselves an unplayable lie—or position ourselves so that our remaining time can be productive, creative and meaningful. Each of us can indeed make the world a little better than it is right now. But we have to be here to do that.

7

What Should I Get Screened For— How and When?

Better health is an individual responsibility,
and it is an important national goal. And it's not all
that difficult to do. When it comes to your health,
even little steps can make a big difference.

—President George W. Bush

Almost all of us buckle up—or we should. Many of us use helmets when biking—or know we should. And almost all of us seek shelter inside during a lightning storm. Why? Because we know that it makes good sense to be safe. Knowledge changes behavior. Knowledge empowers us.

Let me get personal for a moment. I know, on a daily basis, the challenge of treating advanced cancer of the colon and rectum. I know that this disease is curable, preventable and beatable if, and only if, detected early. So I discussed having a colonoscopy with my doctor. We agreed that when I was fifty-five, a screening of the entire colon would be sensible. My Easter dinner that year was a gallon of fluids to clean out my colon for the test the next day. The screening was not a big deal, and all was well. But I had positioned myself to detect a disease that could be fatal.

We all need to reduce our risks, whether it's wearing a helmet

or getting our colons checked, so we can go the distance. We can arm ourselves with knowledge and then take action.

Give Your Doctor a Checkup

Note that in my personal example, I talked with my doctor about what I
should do. Sure, I'm a doctor, but we all need a partner in our own health.
This partnership is not only important, it's critical. That's why I suggest you
check out your doctor before you get a checkup.

After all, you price TV sets before you buy. You shop around for auto-
mobiles. You try on clothes. Why not "try on" a new doctor and see if the
chemistry is right? In this chapter, you'll learn the ins and outs of doctor
shopping—what credentials to look for and how to ask, how to check on
the doctor's reputation and whom to believe—even if your choices are limited by managed care.

You may seek a new doctor for a number of reasons: your doctor moves or
retires, you move and want a medical office closer to where you live, or you
change health plans and might have to choose a doctor from a selected list.

Sometimes you will require a doctor with a particular specialty, such as
when you get pregnant and need an obstetrician and then have a child and
need a pediatrician. Other times, you just want another opinion or are dissatisfied and want better care.

Whatever your reason for seeking a new doctor, you'll want to choose a
physician you trust and with whom you are comfortable.

The best time to choose a doctor is when you *don't* need one. Just like
you don't want to be looking through the yellow pages for a lawyer if you're
arrested, you don't want to be searching for a doctor when you have a medical emergency. Check out the doctor first to make sure the doctor is
licensed in your state, has the training you require and has board certification. You can even find out where the doctor had medical training and in
what specialties.

Here's where to start:

- Ask your family, friends and coworkers if they would recommend their
  doctors and why. These are often reliable sources.
- Community hospitals and large medical centers often have
  "Find-a-Doctor" phone referral centers. These are reasonable places to

begin the journey of finding a health-care provider. However, as the Latin saying goes, *caveat emptor,* "let the buyer beware." Once you and your family have the names of physicians or health-care providers, it certainly would be appropriate to check their credentials.

- Your health plan, whether it's an HMO or PPO or some other alphabet-soup plan, may publish a directory of providers in the plan. This is another list to narrow your search.

- Check with your county or state medical societies. You can access many of the state groups through an association of state medical and osteopathic boards at *www.docboard.org.* Not all states are listed on this site, but if yours is, you can search by name and specialty. Depending on the state, you may be able to find out if there is any disciplinary action pending against a specific doctor.

- Some states have Web sites where you can access any medical professionals who might have disciplinary action pending. Simply because a doctor is being sued does not mean that the physician is not qualified, compassionate and thorough. Some lawsuits are frivolous nuisance claims that in no way reflect the judgment of the provider. The response of patients and how that individual is viewed by the medical community are far more important than a legal judgment, which may have no bearing on his or her skills.

- Conduct a national search through the site of the American Medical Association at *www.ama-assn.org/aps/amahg.htm.* You can search by physician name or medical specialty. To locate a doctor near you, enter your zip code. You'll find out where the doctor trained, his or her specialties, and whether the doctor is board certified.

- Look for a board-certified doctor. Go to the American Board of Medical Specialties at *www.abms.org.* Click "Who's Certified" and follow the form. You may also simply ask the doctor or the office staff or look at the framed certificates on the walls at your current doctor's office.

What board certification means

The kind of specialized training a doctor has had in treating you or your condition does matter. Board certification is a credential or an acknowledgment of expertise that the doctor has taken *and passed* a test on a fundamental body of knowledge. Look for "board certification" in the specialty related to your condition when you are seeking a well-trained physician. This is a prerequisite.

If a doctor is a member of a medical specialty society and has board certification, the doctor may have additional letters following his or her name (an example would be John Doe, M.D., F.A.C.S., meaning Dr. Doe is a Fellow of the American College of Surgeons).

This additional certification assures you that the doctor has demonstrated expertise in a specialty area. **Not every doctor has board certification.** A doctor who does not have board certification may not have taken the "boards"—the certification test. Or may have taken it and failed. However, doctors can be excellent caregivers without board certification.

Credentials—a confusing alphabet soup

Now, how to make some sense out of the bewildering alphabet soup of credentials? Most of us recognize the initials for the M.D. (doctor of medicine) or D.O. (doctor of osteopathy), as well as the Ph.D. (doctor of philosophy) and the R.N. (registered nurse). The P.A. is a physician's assistant, and the N.P. is a nurse practitioner—both highly qualified to work under the guidance of your doctor. You may see a C.N.M. (certified nurse midwife) or F.N.P. (family nurse practitioner). For counseling issues, you may work with an M.S.W. (master of social work) or Psy.D. (doctor of psychology). But a host of other professionals with credentials may play a role in the management of your health.

The physical therapist (P.T.) and the doctor of chiropractic (D.C.) are two kinds of professionals who may indeed provide care for you. If you are not familiar with a caregiver's credentials and area of expertise, it might be appropriate to ask for his or her professional credentials and training. If the practitioner is part of your managed care network, you can almost be assured that he or she has been checked out.

Be warned, however, that some so-called professionals with questionable credentials should not be on your medical-management team.

How can you tell the difference?

Anyone worth working with will readily comply if you ask about certification. If the person you are consulting has no state or national licensure board that has approved this person to practice, you need to be concerned. The beauty of the Internet is that it allows you to go to the organization's Web site and check out the credibility online.

If the practitioner with the unusual credentials expects a large "up front" cash advance, or if the person is practicing in a foreign country, you need to be realistic and have legitimate amounts of suspicion. Framed diplomas or fancy letters after someone's name doesn't give them a free pass to practice on you.

Making the final choice

Your final decision in choosing among doctors who are equally trained may come down to personality and practice style. Choose a doctor who communicates well with you. Make an appointment just to meet a potential new doctor.

Ask (and get satisfactory answers to) these questions before you schedule your appointment:

- Are the office hours and location convenient?
- Who covers for the doctor when he or she is off or after hours?
- Is the office and nursing staff courteous? How hard is it to get an appointment when needed? If urgent?
- Will the doctor be a partner with you in your care?

If you feel comfortable with the doctor after checking out the credentials and training, and after meeting the doctor—with your clothes on— trust your instincts. You've probably found the right partner.

The Doctor Doesn't Always Know Best—You Do

Nationwide polls point to cancer as the number-one health concern. Yet despite our concern for this dreaded disease (and others), we often ignore the risk factors in our lives, choose not to follow cancer-prevention diets and lifestyles, think cancer may be inevitable if we have a strong family history of the disease, or don't know how often to be screened for cancer. All these points were clearly made in a poll taken by the American Cancer Society and the Discovery Health Channel.

Yet the fact remains that heart disease—not cancer—will kill more of us than any other disease. Nonetheless, women fear breast and ovarian cancers and skin cancer far out of proportion to their actual risk of dying of these types of cancer. Men are most concerned about prostate and lung cancers. Yet neither men nor women are as concerned about cancers of the colon and rectum (the third most deadly for both genders) as they should be.

What is the single most important determinant of whether you will develop cancer? If you said family history, you are wrong. It's your age. As you age, your risk increases.

You can't control your age, but you can control another factor that plays a very large part in the development of cancer. Two-thirds of cancer deaths are related to one issue. Would you like to guess? It's lifestyle, especially diet—two practices you can control. Which explains why age and lifestyle should be considered when you discuss your medical history with your doctor. You can reduce your risk with early detection and screening, but how often you need certain tests is still not commonly known.

The American Cancer Society recommends a cancer-related checkup every three years for men and women between twenty and thirty-nine, and every year once you hit forty. Chances are you have never had a specific cancer-related checkup. Read this chapter, use the checklist at the end, and let's change that.

Certainly knowing what to do and doing the right things are two different issues, as we discussed earlier in relation to behavior change. One study in the *Annals of Internal Medicine* looked at information from eighty-one other studies (this is known as a meta-analysis) comparing different ways to get people to have preventive checkups.

The researchers found that preventive checkups increased when physician practices set up separate clinics just for prevention and scheduled specific doctor visits with patients just for prevention. Sometimes staff other than doctors performed screening exams. This would be a nurse practitioner or physician assistant along with nurses.

Another incentive for checkups (or excuses for avoiding them) was financial. If your health plan paid for routine physical exams, chances are you were more likely to get one, according to one study. Or perhaps your plan allowed you to pay a smaller copayment for that visit. Not surprisingly, another study found that adults who had to pay for yearly checkups were less likely to want them, though most in the survey of 1,023 adults said they thought yearly exams were necessary.

At one time in medical history, on a fairly regular basis, many patients underwent a comprehensive screening assessment, which often included dangerous, expensive and inconvenient interventions. I can vividly recall as a young medical student at the University of Michigan caring for executives who were hospitalized for up to five days for stomach x-rays, colon x-rays and a battery of other studies that certainly could have been done on an outpatient basis. I am not being critical. This was the method of medical practice at that time in history.

Today, however, the annual physical exam has been reappraised. A careful history and physical exam generally is the cornerstone of an assessment. Routine blood studies assessing anemia, liver functions, thyroid functions, sugar levels, and levels of cholesterol and triglycerides are very reasonable, based on your age, risk factors and gender. Obviously, to subject a healthy high school or college student to these sorts of assessments would not be appropriate.

Appropriate screening studies such as the mammogram, the colonoscopy and the PSA (a blood test to check for prostate cancer) are reasonable. In general, the "annual physical exam" is much more targeted and much more focused on your needs rather than on an indiscriminate "shotgun approach" subjecting the patient to every new technology.

Early Detection: A Mantra to Follow

A dogma of medicine, which is clearly supported by the literature and by statistics, is that the earlier a condition is detected, the better the probability of a cure and a more positive outcome you will have. Let's suppose an individual has vague chest heaviness or tightness with exertion. This is called angina pectoris (chest pain). If this condition is recognized early, it is conceivable that the patient might have a variety of cardiac assessments clearly defining the problem, and this might be corrected by a bypass procedure or by having a stent inserted into the partially blocked coronary artery.

In other words, early detection of the problem can result in a resolution of the problem with continuation of a relatively normal life for the individual. Now let's look at diabetes. Suppose at the time of an annual physical examination an individual has an elevated blood sugar. By finding this condition early with a simple blood test, this person can make lifestyle changes through diet and exercise, which can be introduced so that the condition can be controlled, and the patient may very well live a relatively normal life.

Consider the situation of a potentially blocked carotid artery. This is an artery in the neck that feeds blood from the heart into the brain. If this artery becomes significantly blocked, the patient may have a stroke resulting in significant disabilities, such as paralysis, blindness or even death. If this abnormality is detected early enough during a physical exam—as the doctor listens to blood flow in neck arteries—we can perform surgical and medical interventions to correct the problem so that the patient's life can be not only saved, but enhanced.

Another example is an unusual metabolic disorder called Addison's disease. (This disease results from a failure in the adrenal glands, which are pyramid-shaped structures sitting on top of each kidney that produce cortisone and a variety of other substances.) If this disease is not detected in its early stages, a minor stress such as the flu or pneumonia can cause death. By detecting this condition early with appropriate routine blood tests, patients can take cortisone or prednisone by mouth and live a relatively normal life.

My take-home message: Early detection for any condition, including cancer, results in most cases in a more favorable outcome than if the condition is not found.

There is no question. We are having a great deal of success in the war against cancer and other dreaded diseases. Today, people are living longer than at any time in history. The successes and the breakthroughs in labs and through clinical trials, however, apply to a very small proportion of cancers. For example, patients with cancers arising from the testicle, which have widely spread, are now curable with chemotherapy, as are some types of lung cancers, especially the small-cell type. Childhood cancers, which were uniformly fatal just a few years ago, are now consistently curable.

Yet for most patients with advanced cancers arising from other areas— the gastrointestinal tract, kidneys, bladder, lung and from the skin via malignant melanoma—the survival is not much different now than it was ten or fifteen years ago. In essence, there have been islands of striking success for some patients, but when we step back to the thirty-thousand-foot view and survey the landscape of patients with far-advanced cancer, the progress has been sluggish.

This underscores the overarching importance of lifestyle issues and early detection to enhance our ability to cure cancers. Half of all cancers are caused by lifestyle choices. A sedentary lifestyle, a high-fat diet, inappropriate exposure to the sun, and obviously tobacco and alcohol account for about half of cancers. Therefore, if you become empowered, proactive and assertive, you can shift the odds from the house to your favor by following some common-sense rules of restricting fats, being physically active, using sunscreen, obviously not smoking and restricting alcohol to a minimum.

Now what about early detection and screening? *Screening* is testing to detect a disease. *Detection*, therefore, is what happens during screening that may prevent you from developing a life-threatening illness by nabbing it in its early and highly curable stages.

Catching the Number-One Killer
(P.S.: It's Not Cancer)

Heart disease and stroke are the nation's number-one killers. So it's no wonder the American Heart Association recommends regular blood pressure checks at least every two years starting at age twenty. But being overweight and obese are also clear risk factors for heart disease. Body mass index (BMI) and waist-to-hip comparisons are also measures to assess obesity, but it seems to me that we can do that by looking in the mirror. Keeping your weight in check can be difficult as age seems to creep up on us around our middles. But reasonable and controlled weight gain into middle-age can be done.

Measuring weight is routine in any doctor's visit. And so is taking your blood pressure. You can also slide into one of those blood pressure stations next time you're in a drugstore. Many people keep a card in their wallets or purses and write down the date and their blood pressures. I recommend it. It's relatively easy to measure and track your own numbers in these areas.

Cholesterol measurement, including the full lipid profile that includes all types of cholesterol (HDL and LDL), is another detection tool the American Heart Association recommends every five years starting at age twenty. This involves drawing a small sample of blood. You don't have to wait for a doctor's appointment to get these numbers. If you attend a health fair at work or in the community, you can also keep track of these numbers yourself. Certainly if these measures are high, you'll want to discuss them with your doctor right away. Diet and exercise can make a dramatic difference for you.

With a family history of heart disease, however, you'll want to track these measures much more frequently and partner with your doctor in monitoring your risks.

The Fatal Four and Life's Madness

Even the casual follower of sports is familiar with the Sweet Sixteen, the Final Four, the Big Dance. This is college basketball's finest hour. A sixty-four-team elimination tournament crowns the national champion of collegiate basketball.

This tournament does not rely on a poll of sportswriters to crown the national champion. There is a clear-cut winner and plenty of losers. The winner climbs the highest peak of college basketball's stardom by hard work, athletic savvy, and by being proactive and assertive.

For the cancer doctor, the Fatal Four are cancers of the lung, breast, colon and prostate. These killers account for more than half of all cancer deaths in the United States. The madness about these cancers is that, in large part, they are preventable, avoidable and curable if detected at an early stage. Like the NCAA champions, we can take steps to increase the probabilities of victories. A guarantee? Of course not. But we can clearly position ourselves to come away with the final victory.

Cancer is the disease the public fears most, which is why screening for cancer is so vital. I'm not downplaying the importance of uncovering a developing glaucoma or high blood sugar, but with cancer the stakes are high. So let's cover cancer detection now and then move toward other conditions that benefit from early detection and treatment.

Which Tests to Have When, and What the Results Mean

The American Cancer Society has made screening recommendations, and I want to walk you through which tests you need, when, and, of course, why. I suggest you use the *cancer worksheets* at the end of this chapter to keep track of the tests you undergo and the results. It would be a good idea to bring your chart with you to your medical appointments. While your doctor should have a record of the tests performed by that medical office—and those results should be in your medical chart—I advise you to be the keeper of the master copy of this information. Charts are misplaced and information misfiled, and you may change doctors to see different specialists.

| **Fecal occult blood test (FOBT) and flexible sigmoidoscopy** | men and women | FOBT every year and flexible sigmoid-oscopy every 5 years, starting at age 50 |

OR

Flexible sigmoidoscopy, every 5 years starting at age 50

OR

Fecal occult blood test every year starting at age 50

OR

Colonoscopy every 10 years starting at age 50

OR

Double-contrast barium enema (DCBE) every 5 years starting at age 50

Cancer of the colon is a major killer in this country. Long-term dietary and population studies strongly hint that a diet high in red meat and a high-fat diet have something to do with the frequency of this disease. Some interesting studies have also indicated that physically active people may decrease their risk of colon cancer. Now why should this be?

It may be related to less contact time between the food we eat and the lining of the colon. Undoubtedly, there are cancer-causing chemicals in what we eat, and by rapidly transporting these materials through the colon, there is a lower frequency of the genetic mutation that may result in cancer.

Fecal occult blood test

At one time, the fecal occult blood test was viewed as the gold standard for the evaluation of cancers of the colon and rectum. The theory went something like this: Cancers would typically bleed and that blood could be detected by smearing a stool specimen on a small piece of cardboard about the size of a credit card. A chemical reaction would then change the color of the card to indicate the possible presence of blood.

Sounds simple enough, but . . . some cancers do not bleed on a regular basis and would be missed by this test. On the other hand, if you had eaten a cheeseburger or taken an aspirin within several days of the test, there could be a false positive. This means that the test was positive, but that positive result did not necessarily mean that cancer was present. The test could be falsely positive because taking some medications like aspirin cause some oozing or bleeding from the intestinal tract.

Even if a repeat test is normal, you might have a nagging anxiety that a serious problem could be missed. This is why we don't consistently recommend the fecal occult blood test. If the test is positive, it usually is repeated. If it is positive a second time, then a colonoscopy typically is recommended. If the test is negative, a colonoscopy may still be recommended if you are at high risk for cancer of the colon or rectum (family history or history of having multiple polyps in the colon). Many doctors continue to use this test but only in conjunction with other assessments.

The stool sample test is not a final analysis. Don't rely on it.

Sigmoidoscopy

Sigmoidoscopy is not a big deal if the procedure is done by an experienced operator. This screening test typically is done by a primary care physician, an internist or a gastroenterologist. To find how experienced the operator is, ask the doctor how many of these procedures he or she does each year. You want someone who does these all the time.

During the procedure, the doctor inserts a flexible, lighted telescope gently into your rectum and into the lower part of your colon specifically to search for abnormalities, especially cancer. Patients are often instructed to drink liberal quantities of fluids twenty-four hours before the procedure and then to use one or two over-the-counter enemas. This consists of a tube, much like a tube of toothpaste, with a small plastic nozzle. The ingredients of the tube are gently squeezed into the rectum to clean out the lining of that organ so that the walls of the colon can be clearly seen.

This procedure can be a bit uncomfortable, but overall it has relatively few risks and often is safely done on an outpatient basis. Most patients are asked to position themselves in the knee-to-chest position in which they are leaning on their elbows and knees as the tube is inserted. Under some circumstances, patients may be lying on their right or left side with their legs flexed as the procedure is being done. In most cases, IV sedation is not needed. The procedure takes about fifteen minutes to check just the lower part of the bowel.

This is an excellent test, but it's not adequate to find a cancer of the colon that may be beyond the reach of the shorter scope. I recommend, instead, a colonoscopy that checks the entire colon.

Colonoscopy

It is not polite dinner conversation to talk about one's colonoscopy or other scoping of the colon and rectum. However, a colonoscopy, while uncomfortable, is not really a big deal and can assure you of at least having a chance for a healthy and well life. In other words, don't wait for symptoms. Ask your doctor about setting up a schedule.

A colonoscopy usually requires some mild IV sedation, takes about thirty to forty-five minutes, and assesses the whole length of the colon. It usually is advocated at age fifty and every ten years after that, though it may be advised starting earlier in life and more frequently for individuals with polyps or a family history of colon cancer.

Thanks to advancing technology making nearly everything "virtual," colleagues at Stanford are testing a virtual colonoscopy. It's not as simple as we'd like it to be, however. Test subjects still have to empty their colons with a day of preparation, and if suspicious polyps are spotted on the series of images taken from the outside of the body, guess what's next? A trip inside with a real colonoscope.

Double-contrast barium enema

Some patients in consultation with their doctors might opt for the double-contrast barium enema instead of a colonoscopy. This is time-consuming and more of a hassle than a colonoscopy. In this procedure, the doctor inserts two tubes into your rectum. One injects barium into your colon and creates a thin layer of barium (this stuff shows up on an x-ray) to coat the lining. Air from the other tube forces the barium into your entire colon. Many patients report that this procedure is uncomfortable. Much like rolling a baking pan to coat it with oil, doctors have to roll you into different positions to be sure the entire lining of the colon is coated.

X-ray images are then taken to view irregularities in the colon lining. You are required to be alert and cooperative—and you must keep the barium in your colon when your greatest urge is to find a bathroom quickly. I opt for colonoscopy.

People who see their doctors for regular preventive care are more likely to have colorectal screening, but only about 20 percent of adults older than age fifty have had a fecal occult blood test in the past year, according to research reported in the *American Journal of Preventive Medicine*. So far fewer have had a colonoscopy, which is appalling considering the high rate of this type of cancer and our ability to deal with it. Insurance—or lack of it—is often a contributing factor.

Digital rectal examination and prostate specific antigen test (PSA)	men age 50+	every year

Prostate cancer was once viewed as a disease of older men in nursing homes. Not now. For some reason, this cancer has become aggressive and virulent and can occur in men in their forties.

Cancer of the prostate is an enormous problem, especially in the African American community. The disease seems to occur among younger individuals in this population group and may be clinically more dangerous. Interesting studies have suggested that if you're physically active, you may decrease the risk of this cancer. Obviously, these leads from population studies are tantalizing and require meticulous study, but I don't think we can ignore some of these preliminary findings.

Virtually every major medical organization now advocates that, starting at age fifty, men should have a yearly digital rectal examination in conjunction with prostate specific antigen (PSA) screening.

Digital rectal examination

The digital rectal examination is a routine part of any physical exam. You should expect it to be part of yours. The rectal exam is performed on both men and women. The doctor inserts a lubricated, gloved finger into your rectum. With gentle pressure, an examination in men is done of the lower rectum as well as the prostate. The procedure has virtually no associated risks. For women, the examination is used to detect any masses or abnormalities in the lower rectum.

Sure, it's mildly uncomfortable, but the treatment for an advanced cancer is much rougher to get through. Some patients are examined while they lie on their backs. Others might be asked to fold into the knee-to-chest position lying on their sides.

As a male, I can understand why patients have little enthusiasm for the digital rectal exam. It is hardly the highlight of my year. When properly done with a fully lubricated and gloved hand and when not done hastily, the procedure is not a great discomfort. However, I clearly know that cancer of the prostate can be a major-league inconvenience to my retirement plans if not detected early. The exam is rarely painful, takes just a short time (perhaps thirty to forty-five seconds), even though it seems like longer. And you get the peace of mind that all is okay.

None of us—men or women—is immune from cancer of the rectum. This is why each of us should expect the annual rectal exam. Less frequently, this exam might detect other potentially serious cancer-related problems. For example, malignant melanoma and skin cancers are sometimes found at the time of the rectal exam. Prior to inserting the gloved and lubricated examining finger, the health-care provider should look at the skin between the buttocks and around the anus for telltale signs of a potentially serious problem. Again, these are very rare but curable cancers if detected early. You are much more likely to detect your own skin cancer on an area you look at more often.

Prostate specific antigen (PSA)

The PSA test is crucial—insist on it. Otherwise, you may not have to worry about retirement. PSA is a chemical that can be detected in the blood through a simple blood test. Depending on the specific method used, the range of normal may be from 0 up to 4. If the test is higher than 4, that does not necessarily mean that cancer is present.

As men get older, the prostate typically increases in size. The larger the prostate, the higher the normal number can be for the PSA. However, if the PSA continues to increase, that's when we doctors get concerned that the gland is harboring a cancer. As with most medical decisions, care has to be tailored to you.

We now know that African Americans have a strikingly high rate of cancer of the prostate. Therefore, if an African American man is forty-two and his PSA level is 4—with 4 being the upper limit of normal—then multiple biopsies certainly need to be considered. Generally, the high-risk man would start with a PSA analysis at age forty.

When the level is 4, we closely monitor the situation and worry when it gets to 8 and much higher. Another factor is the rate of increase. In other words, if it takes two or three years for the level to go from 4 to 8, that is much less worrisome than if the level goes from 4 to 8 in a few months. Again, no universal "cookbook" exists, and these laboratory tests can be interpreted only within the context of the individual patient, his age, the rate of increase, family history, and racial and ethnic background.

A biopsy of the prostate normally involves taking multiple samples of tissue from a specific area of abnormality. If we can detect a nodule, or can see a nodule by using ultrasound imaging, we'll get samples from that area of the prostate. However, a very challenging situation is the man who has a rising PSA and a normal gland on physical examination and a normal gland on ultrasound assessment. In these situations, the worry is that there are some microscopic cancer cells that cannot be seen or detected but are clearly present and are producing the elevation of the PSA. In this circumstance some men are advised to undergo biopsies in which samples are randomly taken of the gland. Usually, before the biopsies are obtained, a topical anesthetic is injected into the gland to decrease the discomfort.

Most men tolerate this procedure reasonably well, but there is always concern for blood in the urine and significant discomfort (our way of saying "pain") in a minority of men who undergo biopsies. Tissue taken from these samples is examined under a microscope for cancer.

Most men who already have prostate cancer advocate routine PSA blood testing because they know that early diagnosis will reduce death and improve quality of life. They've been there and done that and want their own friends and sons to be vigilant. This was the conclusion of a study that appeared in the *British Medical Journal*.

For high-risk individuals such as African American men and those with a strong positive family history, screenings should be started in the forties. Early detection means cure.

This cancer is especially devastating because impotence and incontinence may result, not from the cancer, but from the treatment. Because many men live for years after the diagnosis, quality of life becomes a big issue. We really do not fully understand which men should have their prostates removed as a means of treatment. Some men may have a quiet, smoldering form of the disease for decades. They don't require aggressive treatment. For them, a watch-and-wait approach may be sensible, but the risk is that the cancer could become more serious during this period.

If cancer is present, you should seek another opinion from a specialist in cancer and urology so that you are comfortable making your final decision. Yes, that's your decision.

Obviously, no test or exam is foolproof, but a normal rectal exam and a normal PSA are highly reassuring that cancer of the prostate is not present at that time.

Now a word about a cancer that men don't talk about. Testicular cancer is the most common cancer in men between ages twenty and thirty-four. That is why each testicle needs to be examined during the physical. Every man should examine his own testicles monthly anyway. Don't ignore a painless mass or an aching discomfort in the scrotum or groin. If you have an area of concern, a testicular ultrasound test may be done. This involves placing a small device (it looks like a microphone) on the testicle. The ultrasound images are then reviewed for cancerous masses or areas of suspicion.

Do these tests save lives?

You may have read about recent studies purporting that aggressive screening and treatment do not reduce deaths from prostate cancer. But, when it's your prostate and your future, do you really want to skip a simple blood test and manual exam? (The same thing goes for mammograms and breast self-exams.)

The United States Preventive Services Task Force has taken a neutral position on whether the digital rectal exam and PSA are useful in preventing illness and death. But from a practicing physician's perspective, these are routine and standard and part of the normal evaluation of a patient. Let me explain. It is clear that the earlier that a cancer is diagnosed, the better the outcome. I know of no cancer in which an advanced form of the disease has a higher cure rate than the early form of the disease. In other words, early detection gives the patient the best chance of long-term benefit.

The digital rectal examination is one attempt to detect a cancer of the rectum at its early stage. If the physician feels an abnormality, this is sometimes followed up with the flexible sigmoidoscopic examination or a colonoscopy. This is an important part of the physical examination, especially if the patient has rectal or anal complaints or concerns.

Fully recognizing the controversy about the PSA, it is fair to state that most clinicians see the value of this test. This is especially important for high-risk groups for cancer of the prostate (African Americans, individuals with a strong positive family history). If the blood test is significantly elevated, this might indicate the need for a biopsy to find the cancer at an early stage.

Now here comes the uneasy news. Is it possible that the patient's cancer in the prostate can remain quiescent or dormant for many years before causing any problems? And the answer is maybe. This occurs when a physician—and patient—take a wait-and-see philosophy. For some men, it is unsettling to know that there is a cancer present and not do something about it. For those men, surgery is reasonable. The wait-and-see philosophy does not have strong advocates, and there is a tendency among most patients and health-care providers to instead consider surgery or radiation for these early-stage cancers of the prostate.

Bottom line: Although controversy exists among the experts, the weight of evidence and the standard of medical practice in most communities is for the digital rectal examination and the PSA to be performed annually, or more frequently, based on the patient's age and risks for either cancer of the prostate or cancer of the rectum.

Pap test and pelvic examination   women, age 18+

All women who are, or have been, sexually active or have reached age 18 should have an annual Pap test and pelvic examination. After a woman has had three or more consecutive satisfactory normal annual examinations, the Pap test may be performed less frequently at the discretion of the physician.

Cancer of the cervix is a preventable and curable cancer, if detected early. With positive lymph nodes, meaning the cancer has spread, the chance of cure decreases dramatically—often vanishing. The treatment often involves a combination of chemotherapy and radiation. The routine Pap smear is the best way to eliminate the difficult treatment required by this type of tumor.

Expect a Pap test and pelvic examination as part of your annual checkup. During the Pap test, a small brush is inserted into the opening of the uterus. Cells are scraped off, placed on a glass slide or into a small bottle, and looked at under a microscope. As part of the procedure, a physical exam is done of the female organs and rectum.

At one time, a woman would undergo a routine Pap smear and pelvic exam virtually every year regardless of her age. It is now becoming clear that as individuals reach their seventies and eighties this recommendation needs to be reevaluated. If a woman is not sexually active and has had no previously abnormal Pap smears, to discontinue the annual Pap smear in the seventies certainly seems reasonable.

But again, many of these recommendations need to be applied to a specific patient. For example, if a woman in her thirties has multiple sexual partners and is sexually active, yearly Pap smears and pelvic exams are certainly appropriate. On the other hand, if a woman is celibate and does not have any significant gynecologic history, performing Pap smears and pelvic exams at a less frequent interval certainly makes good sense.

Older women should be alert to the significance of bleeding from the uterus after menopause. A cancer of the uterus may first become evident by bleeding from the vagina. Again, early detection gives far better odds of a cure than detecting a cancer that has spread. In most cases, bleeding is not serious. But if it continues, it does need attention. Expect your doctor to recommend an endometrial tissue sample (biopsy), especially if you experience postmenopausal bleeding.

A scraping of the lining of the uterus (for an endometrial uterine biopsy) is an office procedure with low risks. Occasionally, cancer cells from the ovary may be detected this way. Again, early detection raises the odds of long-term cure. Don't ignore your body's signals that something's wrong.

A vaccine to protect against cervical cancer is on the horizon for a whole generation of young women. It will undoubtedly be particularly important in underserved populations in this country and throughout the world for whom cervical cancer unfortunately remains a leading cause of death. The idea of a vaccine against cancer is enticing and shows the value of tenacious research. Because some cervical cancers develop from exposure to the human papillomavirus (often a sexually transmitted disease), this may be a model for attacking some virus-triggered cancers, but a vaccine is not applicable to the big killers: lung, breast, colon and prostate cancers.

Breast self-examination	women age 20+ monthly starting at age 20
Clinical breast examination	annual, starting at age 40 (prior to mammography)
Mammography	annual, starting at age 40

As every woman reading this book knows, breast cancer is a national catastrophe. Approximately one woman in eight or nine will develop this cancer. The emotional and psychological impact of breast cancer is profound. Spectacular advances in the hormonal treatment of breast cancer have opened great possibilities for long-term benefit. However, we need to recognize that, as with colon cancer, early detection is the key.

Breast self-exam

Every woman knows these self-exams aren't foolproof, but we all know you need to do it every month. Some studies have recently suggested that the breast self-exam is not necessary. In fact, headlines such as "Study finds no evidence that teaching breast self-examination saves lives" make me cringe. A study in the *Journal of the National Cancer Institute* found that women who examined their breasts found lumps that turned out to be fine after a small surgical procedure. The bottom line for the researchers was that these unnecessary biopsies added to already high health-care costs. What am I missing here? If that's your breast and your lump, wouldn't you want to find it and find out what it was?

The researchers also concluded that doctors should not spend time teaching women how to conduct a breast self-exam but should spend more time educating women about breast cancer symptoms—such as a lump or nipple discharge—and spend more time on the clinical breast exam they conduct in the office. Again, what am I missing here? Whether the woman finds the lump or the doctor finds a lump, we still don't know what it is without further testing.

Naturally, breast-cancer prevention groups are up in arms, and I cannot blame them. Until this controversy settles out, I think a woman should be proactive and assertive in asking for instructions on breast self-exam. We are clearly learning that the physical exam alone is not adequate to detect cancers, so this technique must be used in concert with mammograms. These recommendations continue to be a "moving target." Web sites such as Mayo Clinic (*www.MayoClinic.com*) and the American Cancer Society (*www.cancer.org*) are excellent resources to get the most up-to-date information in this area.

A revealing survey by the Susan G. Komen Breast Cancer Foundation found that young women in their twenties and thirties are not performing monthly breast self-exams because most don't think they are at risk.

Certainly being a woman and growing older are risk factors, but breast cancer remains the leading cause of cancer for women in this younger age
range, too. Sadly, women diagnosed this young often have a more aggressive form of the disease.

Another survey finding from the Komen study was even more surprising:
40 percent of young women incorrectly thought mammograms *prevented*
breast cancer rather than screened for the disease. This figure is disturbing
and reflects much misunderstanding and misinformation surrounding the
management and the diagnosis of breast cancer. A mammogram is a diagnostic, fact-finding approach to detect cancers but certainly does not prevent disease. We in the medical-care community have a responsibility to
make certain that patients understand why tests are performed. We obviously have work to do here.

Primary-care doctors and ob/gyns taking care of these women have a
great opportunity to provide education in the form of eye-to-eye counseling, materials such as videos and shower cards showing the self-exam techniques, and Web site referrals so patients can learn the importance of this
technique and how to do it in the privacy of their homes.

Mammography

Mammograms can detect a cancer the size of a grain of rice and can
offer a high chance of cure. My female patients tell me the anticipation of
having a mammogram creates an enormous amount of anxiety. The reason
is obvious.

Every woman knows what the radiologist is looking for, and every woman
dreads the possibility of a malignant tumor being detected in her breast. I
almost always ask patients about the level of discomfort from the procedure. In general, I am hearing that the discomfort largely depends on the
skill and the sensitivity of the technician performing the test.

For reasons that I do not think that any of us really understands, the procedure can go very smoothly in some women without much discomfort, but
in others it can be very uncomfortable. The size and contour of the breasts
do not seem to make a difference in comfort level. One factor makes the
test somewhat bearable. The discomfort only lasts for a few minutes, and
most patients are able to understand the importance of "bearing with" the
compression of the breasts while the test is performed.

Although some controversy exists regarding the schedule for screening mammograms, the American Cancer Society now recommends starting with a mammogram at age forty, then every year through age seventy or seventy-five and even later. Women should have an annual mammogram in conjunction with a clinical breast examination. In this procedure, your doctor will carefully examine each breast and palpate or feel the tissue as you sit, again while you lie down, and also with your hands on your hips. He or she will pay careful attention to the lymph nodes in the areas behind the collarbone and armpit (axilla).

Here's why the lymph nodes are so important. The larger the cancer, the greater chance the lymph nodes are contaminated. If the breast cancer is detected early, it is highly curable. With lymph nodes involved, chances for cure drop.

If the cancer is small (an inch or less), then cure rates at twenty years may be almost 90 percent. But if the cancer is four inches or larger, the average time for the cancer to come back is only four months, and almost none are cured. Even one involved lymph node dramatically reduces the chances for cure. For patients with one to three nodes involved, the ten-year survival rate is about 50 percent.

Don't rely on the "system" to send you reminder notices about your next mammogram. It's up to you to remember when you had a mammogram and to schedule another. Absolutely begin screening with these simple x-rays by age forty. A clinical breast examination is done by a doctor or nurse practitioner.

Men, too, can get breast cancer. (However, women never get prostate cancer!) A painless lump or nipple discharge needs to be assessed with a mammogram and a careful physical exam. A biopsy is often done to determine the diagnosis. About 30 percent of these men have a positive family history of breast cancer in either males or females. That's why doctors should ask about your family tree.

Health counseling and   men and women age 20+
cancer checkup

Examinations every three years from age 20 to 39 and annually after age 40. The cancer-related checkup should include examination for cancers of the thyroid, testicles, ovaries, lymph nodes, oral cavity and skin, as well as health counseling about tobacco, sun exposure, diet and nutrition, risk factors, sexual practices, and environmental and occupational exposures.

We know good habits must be formed and reinforced early. That's why the American Cancer Society recommends a cancer checkup and health counseling starting as young as age twenty. I've given detailed information about the major cancer screenings. Now here's what a doctor is looking for in examining the rest of your body in these sort-of-annual physicals:

- **Thyroid:** If your thyroid gland (it's at the bottom of your neck, in front) is enlarged, a simple biopsy with a needle can determine if a cancer is present. With early detection, you have a high chance for cure.

- **Lymph nodes:** If they are enlarged, it could mean lymphoma or Hodgkin's disease (cancers of the lymph nodes or bone marrow). But most swollen nodes are not cancerous.

- **Mouth:** Simple inspection of your tongue, palate, lips and cheeks can detect an early and curable cancer. Often, dental hygienists perform this routinely while cleaning your teeth and are the first to spot oral cancers, especially among smokers and those who chew tobacco.

- **Skin:** There are specific ways to tell if a mole is malignant once it is found—by you or your physician. If it is removed early, the chance of a cure is virtually assured. If not found early, you may face major surgery and possibly need toxic and aggressive chemotherapy with or without radiation.

For me, now in my late fifties, I have a yearly checkup with a superb family doctor who listens and is in a partnership with me. My physical exam includes the rectal and prostate and testicular assessment, a PSA blood test, and other routine blood tests. Each three to five years, I have either a flexible sigmoidoscopy exam or colonoscopy. With newer technologies that include thin, flexible scopes and better-trained physicians, these tests are not a big deal. How do I know? Because I have asked for them myself. The biggest hassle is drinking the liquid or taking the pills to clean out the bowel before the procedure. In the days of the rigid scopes, strolling through your colon was a big deal. Today it is not.

When Screening Is Not Enough—The Lungs

When it comes to lung cancer, there's no mystery. What a national and global catastrophe! Lung cancer is the number-one cause of cancer-related deaths in men and women. It accounts for a third of all cancer deaths. And it is preventable because smoking is the "smoking gun" in almost all cases.

The progression is simple: The younger the age you start to smoke, the more cigarettes you smoke over your soon-to-be-abbreviated lifetime, the greater your risk. But it is never too late to stop. Studies show that after a number of years without smoking, the risk of lung cancer decreases until eventually your risk approaches that of a nonsmoker.

By the time a chest x-ray shows lung cancer, it has been present for at least four to six years and contains a billion cancer cells. So early detection really does not apply to lung cancer, and you can't rely on a chest x-ray. Fortunately, early work with the spiral CT scan may show lung cancers earlier, but it's still too early to tell if screening all smokers will catch lung cancers earlier and lower the death rate.

So how do we normally detect lung cancer? Our patients show up coughing bloody phlegm, with shortness of breath, pneumonia, weight loss, bone pain, hoarseness, and shoulder or arm pain. And if the cancer has already spread to the brain—because lung cancer is highly aggressive—a patient may feel weakness in an arm or leg, suffer confusion, and have headaches or seizures.

Few advanced lung cancer patients live longer than a year. But miracles do indeed happen. One of my patients had a highly aggressive and virulent form of lung cancer, which was moved away with treatment from major structures around the heart and aorta. He had a stormy postoperative course but has made a full recovery.

The patient shared with me the following story: He had been ill for several weeks and visited a physician in rural Wyoming, where he lives. He was then referred to a major city hospital in Wyoming where he was clearly told that he was "a dead man." At that point the patient sought another opinion, not from a physician but from a minister. This minister made a claim: "I can pray the spots off a leopard." At the same time, the patient was advised to see a physician at the request of the minister. With the support of the minister and appropriate medical therapy, he has continued to do well. The patient has a very realistic outlook, recognizes that his cancer will undoubtedly reoccur, but at least for the present time, together they prayed the spots off the leopard and he is cancer-free.

The madness about cancer is that we have the tools, techniques and education to dramatically enhance the health, wellness and quality of life for ourselves, family, friends and neighbors. As with the NCAA basketball tournament, we need to position ourselves for a victory. We need to be proactive, assertive and informed, and we need to take charge. To rely on the medical profession or to rely on someone else to do it for us is not the ticket to the Big Dance. It is the ticket to the Big Heartache. The choice is ours. The ball is in our court.

Are You Ever Too Old for Screening?

Doctors can agree on when to start health screening, such as routine mammograms, but we can't agree on when to stop screening. Some doctors think age seventy-five may signal the end of routine screenings for breast, colon and cervical cancer. After all, they reason in the journal of *Effective Clinical Practice,* an older person may suffer more harm from a false positive and surgery. A ninety-year-old man with a small prostate tumor will die from something else, not prostate cancer. They see no economic benefit in terms of years of life saved (of course, they're not talking about your father).

Now comes the tension between experts caring for the individual patient and experts responsible for national health policy. A middle road exists: Each patient needs to be viewed as an individual, not as a cold statistic or a blip on some economist's spreadsheet.

I assessed an eighty-three-year-old woman who looked more fit and was more vital than some of my neighbors who are twenty-five years younger. We need to acknowledge that we are living longer than any generation in history (for a good reason), and if a woman is married and sixty-five, she may well live to be over ninety years old. Now if the screening test is painful, difficult to prepare for (as some think preparing for a colonoscopy is difficult), and if the patient has no complaints and a negative family history, then fine. Forgo the procedure. But mammograms in a woman who may live to one hundred do not seem unreasonable.

Think about it. People are living longer because we're screening and catching that high blood pressure, the precancerous lesion, the tiny skin cancer—or I'd sure like to think so.

But this decision is yours. As a general rule, if you have an anticipated life expectancy of ten more years, continuing your annual screening may be a reasonable choice.

WHO IS BEST AT DETECTING SKIN CANCER?

Generally, you, not your doctor or a nurse, are the first to detect a malignant melanoma (a deadly form of skin cancer) when it occurs on your skin. Not surprisingly, women more frequently detect a malignant melanoma than do men. This is consistent with many studies documenting that women are the drivers of health-care consumerism, and it is the woman who often makes health-care decisions for the entire family.

So don't wait for an annual physical exam to see if the doctor spies something unusual. If you think a mole looks different in some way or a freckle is changing, see your doctor right away. When it comes to your family, it sure doesn't hurt to give each other a once-over. Here's why.

In about 10 to 15 percent of people with malignant melanoma, the first indication of a problem arises from the metastatic disease rather than from the primary or what is known as the occult primary site. Let me explain.

A fairly common scenario is that a person awakens one day and finds a lump under the armpit. A biopsy of the lymph node shows malignant melanoma. In around 90 percent of people, a primary malignant melanoma can be detected in the vicinity of the armpit. This was the "mother cancer" from whence arises the rogue cell that seeds into the lymph nodes. These primary sites are what we all want to detect early—long before it decides to move anywhere else in your body.

But in the other 10 percent of people, we never find the primary neoplasm (or mole). We suspect that there was a primary at some point in time, but then the primary dries up, falls off or is somehow devoured by the body's immune system. However, this process does not occur until after a bizarre cell has broken loose from the primary site and has set up a beachhead in a lymph node.

(continued on following page)

A swollen lymph node may not be the first sign. In some people, the first evidence of malignant melanoma is a seizure. An appropriate scan of the brain then documents metastatic malignant melanoma and a primary site is never found. At this point, finding the primary site is not relevant. The patient is faced with a far-advanced disease somewhere else, such as the brain, bone, liver or spinal cord.

Here are some other examples of what we call the "unknown primary malignant melanoma" that we see on a fairly consistent basis:

- A woman who has a routine Pap smear and pelvic exam shows evidence of a vaginal/rectal malignant melanoma. This obviously is not an area exposed to the sun and does emphasize how little we really do understand about these tumors.
- An individual has a lump under the skin that seems to be innocent, but a biopsy (tissue sample) shows malignant melanoma.
- Someone who coughs up blood has a chest x-ray that is abnormal. A biopsy of the lung indicates metastatic malignant melanoma in the lungs without any obvious primary site.

In other words, a lump or bump or a spot or a swelling that is relatively new and without obvious explanation (you don't remember hitting it accidentally or falling and being injured) certainly could be a metastatic deposit of malignant melanoma even when the primary malignant melanoma is not detected.

Have I made my point about screening? About knowing your body and knowing when something is different? A few minutes in front of the mirror may be the cheapest medical test you'll ever have.

I just heard about a company that will take digital pictures of your body, about fifty, and store them on a CD-ROM. The idea is to make a photographic record of your skin for comparison purposes either annually or whenever you suspect a new mole has appeared. Frankly, nothing will replace the skilled eye of your doctor, preferably a dermatologist, who can make a similar assessment. And with the simplicity of digital photography these days, you could do this yourself and keep your own records.

Other Screening Tests: Well Worth Paying For— Or Not Worth the Time and Money?

You may have heard about certain other screening tests—other than the standard tests recommended by the American Cancer Society and American Heart Association. Some of these can be useful in certain circumstances, depending on your family history. Some of them may well be worth paying for (because your insurance company may not cover them). Others may not be a good investment of your time and money. But let's look at some options.

Genetic testing for colon cancer

Some families are at an especially high risk for cancers arising from the colon and rectum. If you have a first-degree relative (mother, father, brother, sister) who has had this disease or if there are family members with cancer of the colon or rectum occurring at relatively young ages (younger than forty), you may be at risk.

Genetic tests can be performed on your blood to identify abnormalities in genetic material, which might signal that you're prone to developing cancer. However, as with most tests and medicine, the findings are not absolutely foolproof. Sometimes the results can be misleading. And detecting an abnormal gene in your DNA does not necessarily mean that you will develop cancer.

There is another problem: You can imagine the psychological impact of being told that you have a defective gene and that you might develop cancer of the colon. That's the dark side to genetic testing. If a genetic test is "positive" and that leaves you at risk for developing cancer, what does this mean for your employability and insurability? Would you miss out on a job because your employer finds out you may be at risk? Would an insurance company deny you coverage for health or life insurance based on this genetic test?

So what are some practical suggestions?

Genetic testing is a very personal decision. Some people have a need to know, and if that is your situation, a blood test would be reasonable—as long as you fully recognize the limitations of that test. From a practical standpoint, screening colonoscopy starting at age forty or ten years before the youngest member of the family developed colon cancer would be smart. But in general, most of us who are not at high risk for colorectal cancer should start screening at age fifty.

Endometrial (uterine) biopsy, transvaginal ultrasound, CA-125 testing for endometrial and ovarian cancers

If you're a woman beyond menopause and you have vaginal bleeding, then your doctor may discuss with you a scraping of the lining of the uterus. This material is then looked at under the microscope to see if it contains cancer. This procedure, an endometrial or uterine biopsy, is typically performed in the doctor's office. It's relatively safe and is an important test to discuss with your doctor.

A transvaginal ultrasound consists of a small probe somewhat like a thermometer being inserted into the vagina. The probe is then gently positioned through the cervix, which is the opening leading into the uterus itself. This is an outpatient/office procedure and typically is not any more uncomfortable than having a routine Pap smear and pelvic examination—so my female patients tell me.

The images obtained from the ultrasound look like radar images and can help determine if there are masses or abnormalities in the pelvic area. As with many imaging interventions, this test likewise is not foolproof. But if a woman has symptoms such as pain, bloating or fullness, and if there is a family history of female cancers, this test is reasonable.

CA-125 (the CA stands for carbohydrate antigen) is a substance found in blood that acts as a marker or a barometer or a "surrogate" for some types of cancers. It was thought that an elevated CA-125 level might indicate a woman may have ovarian cancer. However, the test is not perfect and is not always specific for cancer. Some women may have an elevated CA-125 but may not have a malignant disease. But the test is still used to monitor whether chemotherapy is working to contain certain female cancers.

Now what about getting the CA-125 "just to make certain that everything is okay"? The problem with this approach is that the levels may be minimally elevated, and CT scans or ultrasound examinations of the abdomen and pelvis may not confirm or rule out that a cancer exists. Then what do you do? We can imagine the anxiety of this situation. Therefore, if you do not have specific symptoms and if your family history is not overwhelmingly positive, these types of tests typically are not done on a routine basis.

Early mammograms for breast cancer

One thing is clear—mammograms are detecting breast cancers at a far more curable stage than at any time in history. It is not uncommon to see breast cancers that are about the size of a match head being detected on the mammogram.

But when mammograms are performed in women younger than forty, the results are sometimes difficult to interpret. Younger women's breasts are normally dense, and the mammograms are not as reliable as they are for older women. With age, the density becomes less intense, and fat becomes more apparent on the mammogram. The contrast between the fat in the breast tissue and the normal breast glands allows for more accurate detection of significant abnormalities.

Generally, though, most professional medical groups agree that a yearly mammogram should be performed starting at age forty.

Genetic mutation–linked cancers (BRCA1, BRCA2)

Within the last decade, scientists identified genes BRCA1 and BRCA2 that, when normal, facilitate the repair of DNA. This protects against the development of cancer. On the other hand, when these genes are abnormal or defective, risk of cancer is strikingly higher. Some studies suggest that when these genes are abnormal, women may have a 56 to 87 percent lifetime chance of developing breast cancer and a 20 to 60 percent chance of developing cancer of the ovary.

As with other forms of genetic testing, the analysis of chromosomes for these defective genes has far-reaching implications. Here is the dilemma: If I as a woman have an abnormal gene, does this mean my other family members should be tested? Even if my gene is abnormal, I may not necessarily develop breast cancer, but my risks are high.

If a woman is at high risk for these cancers because she has many first-degree family members having this condition, genetic testing is reasonable. But I suggest you need to ask a very piercing question: If I test abnormal, what do I do with the results?

In this case, some women, in order to give themselves the very best chance of long-term survival, have opted to have both breasts removed. Studies now demonstrate that this is a reasonable option for some women who are especially concerned about the probability of developing breast cancer.

As another option, if the test is positive, a woman can work with her doctor to develop a plan for careful surveillance in terms of yearly mammograms, prompt biopsies of suspicious lumps or bumps, and the importance of both a professional breast exam and careful training in breast self-exams.

Low-dose spiral CT scan for lung cancer

Lung cancer has clearly reached epidemic proportions in the Western world and is now the leading cause of cancer deaths among women as well as men. The CT scan "slices" the body much like a loaf of bread and can detect nodules far smaller than can be detected on a routine chest x-ray.

Early studies have suggested that lung cancers can be detected at a more curable stage by using the spiral CT scan. However, we do not yet know if this technique will provide long-term benefit for groups of patients. One of the concerns with this technique is detecting small shadows and spots, which are completely harmless but still require ongoing surveillance. We do not know which of these spots and shadows might become cancer. We also do not know how frequently follow-up studies should be performed.

You can understand the anxiety of having a routine screening with a spiral CT scan only to find many small shadows. Some of these may or may not be cancer. This can provoke tremendous anxiety, especially because the medical community at this point does not yet know the best way to follow up with these abnormalities.

Lung cancer is clearly a preventable disease. Smoking is, of course, the leading cause, and never smoking or stopping smoking dramatically reduces anyone's chance of developing lung cancer. Compare that with colon cancer, where the risks are not clearly linked to environmental agents such as cigarette smoke. What is a practical resolution of this dilemma?

If you are at high risk in terms of having a long history of smoking multiple packs of cigarettes per day and have specific symptoms such as cough, shortness of breath, weight loss or coughing up blood that may suggest a potential cancer, the newest high-tech imaging, the CT scan, is certainly reasonable. But as a routine test, we simply don't have the data at hand to recommend its use, despite what you may hear on afternoon talk shows.

Percent-free PSA tests

Prostate-specific antigen (PSA) is a material detected in the blood, which is produced by the prostate gland. The level of PSA in the blood can be high if a man has a harmless enlargement of the prostate gland. But PSA can also be high if a man has cancer of the prostate.

The most widely used PSA test (a blood test) measures the chemical that is bound to a variety of proteins, as well as those that circulate "free" in the bloodstream. Scientists are trying to determine if there is a value of the free-PSA that would help identify those men at greater risk for cancer of the prostate. Studies have been performed among large populations of men suggesting that measuring the percent-free PSA is a helpful technique when the total PSA level is between 2.5 and 10. Men with a total PSA level of 2.5 to 4 with less than 25 percent being "free" can decide whether to undergo a biopsy or wait until the total PSA level exceeds 4. When the level is 4, we monitor closely and worry when it gets to 8 and much higher. Some studies have looked at ratios of the free to the total PSA as providing some guidance. However, in the individual person, various ratios and the amount of the free-PSA provide general guidelines but should not be rigidly followed.

If a man is African American, for example, or if he has a strong family history of cancer of the prostate and there is a suspicious nodule on the prostate, a biopsy typically is recommended regardless of the value of the free-PSA or the total PSA. In other words, we need to understand that the decision for biopsy is complex. It can only be made by understanding the patient himself, his family history, the results of the physical examination, the results of various blood tests and also images of the prostate such as those obtained by an ultrasound of the gland.

The shopping-center full-body scan

Technology can be a wondrous thing. Or not.

It is now becoming fashionable for companies to set up in shopping centers with mobile PET scanners and mobile CT scanners and mobile MRI scanners. These are marvelous high-tech imaging techniques that can detect problems long before they become significant or meaningful. And that's the problem.

Let's suppose we scan one hundred individuals. Almost all of them, if they are adults, will have some spots and shadows on their lungs, for example, which almost never turn out to be cancer. But once we know "something is there," these suspicious areas will need to be followed up, and that means more expensive tests, more anxiety and more inconvenience for the patient.

With a high-tech scan, the "worried well" have opened up Pandora's box and will never be able to get it closed again.

The scanners can see abnormalities, but they can't tell us what they are. So at some point, the patient may become increasingly uneasy about these spots, and a major operation may be necessary to check it out. Mayo Clinic studies have documented that patients will undergo extensive surgery, which obviously is life-threatening, to remove some harmless spots that never would have caused problems.

Therefore, we need ongoing studies to really determine if these shopping-center scans are of any value or if they are simply detecting problems that would never pose any threat to the individual. Worse yet, someone who undergoes a scan and comes out fine may be tempted to skip a regular physical exam for cholesterol and blood pressure testing and other key blood work that the scans don't evaluate.

Our current system of screening works. High-tech scans are not always helpful and can be harmful, especially for relatively healthy people who have no symptoms. If you decide to undergo extensive additional, high-tech scans, you will want to decide up front what you will do about those shadows and spots, if any are detected. Surely, you seek a "clean bill of health," but as we become more sophisticated in peeking inside the human body, we have the unfortunate ability to create more anxiety about the unknown.

Let's Get Physical

The executive physical—it's a highly prized perk for corporate execs, but you can have one too, even if you don't run General Motors. I've asked my colleagues to explain the real "ins and outs" of the popular executive physical conducted at the Clinic. I talked with Dr. Philip T. Hagen in the Department of Preventive Medicine and Dr. Donald D. Hensrud, also in the Department of Preventive Medicine, who heads the Executive Health Plan Program.

Among the CEO crowd, appointment times for these physicals are scheduled a year ahead. But you don't have to wait. You can get the same high-level care from your doctor if you know what to ask for and insist that your doctor partner with you in your care.

How often? Most of us should have periodic health exams during our twenties, thirties and forties, if all is normal. By "periodic," I hope you will be guided by the screening tests outlined in this chapter and by your own sense of comfort—not by how often your insurance company will pay. Once you're past age fifty, you'll need to see your doctor yearly for some screening tests and every few years for others and then yearly after age sixty.

What to Insist On at Your Next Physical

Your medical history

The medical history (which includes your family health history) generally begins with questions like this:

- How are things going?
- What is it that concerns you?
- What are you worried about?
- What brings you to see us today?

I've come to realize that it's the second or third concern the patient mentions, in some circumstances, that is the most significant one. It's my experience that patients don't always know which of their complaints are the most serious. I may be much more concerned about a patient who casually mentions sudden headaches than about the weight gain that causes them the greatest distress.

When you see your doctor, I advise you to focus on two or three key issues such as chest pain, shortness of breath or weight loss rather than waste lots of time on issues that might not be so significant, such as thinning of hair or wrinkles. Now please understand, I don't want you to ignore these concerns, but they may be less significant than the first three. Mention the big ones first.

Think through when your problem began. Tell your doctor what makes it better or worse. These clues will all add up.

Bring a list of all medications you are taking, including prescription drugs, vitamins, minerals, herbs, supplements, nasal sprays, patches—everything. Know the dose you are taking and how often you take the medication. Sometimes it's easier to dump all your medications in a bag and bring them with you. The smart thing, however, is to keep a written record on a file card and keep this card with you (in a wallet or purse) at all times. Such a practice could be lifesaving if you find yourself in a real-life episode of *ER*.

Any medication can produce *side effects,* which are undesirable results from ingredients in the medication. Some are tolerable, such as dry mouth, or unacceptable, such as increased liver damage or heart palpitations. *Interactions,* on the other hand, occur when two or more active ingredients in substances you are taking affect each other. It's the interaction effect that concerns doctors and pharmacists when patients mix prescription drugs and herbals, for example. Herbals can increase or decrease the effects of some medications when used together. At highest risk for interactions are people with chronic conditions, such as stroke, high blood pressure, diabetes and heart disease. Your physical exam may be an ideal time to discuss if you even need to continue taking certain medications.

If you're presenting certain symptoms when you visit the doctor, it will be important for the doctor to rule out or rule in interactions as causes. Even substances you might consider harmless can cause problems, so let your doctor know about it. Here are two examples:

- Ginseng may interfere with a blood thinner you are taking to prevent stroke. It also lowers blood sugar in people who take medicine for diabetes. Even ginseng tea can cause drug–herbal interactions.
- Garlic supplements can change the results of your blood-clotting tests. People who take arthritis pain medications may also be at risk for bruising by taking garlic. And garlic may increase the effect of blood sugar–lowering drugs for those who take diabetes medications. Garlic cooked in foods becomes inactivated because of the heat, so it's fine. Interactions can occur with fresh garlic and concentrated supplements.

It's also important to fill the doctor in on what you do for a living, your hobbies, your social ties and family responsibilities. Everything you say (whether the doctor asks you directly or not) gives the doctor a picture of you.

I recently had the opportunity of seeing a woman who had a very stressful job in a high-tech company. She took an early buy-out and had a wonderful first two years of retirement. She and her husband then bought into a family-run business—and the nightmare began. Following a very contentious interchange with some unpleasant family members, our patient developed two hours of crushing chest pain, was rushed to the hospital, and underwent a complete battery of cardiac assessments that indicated no muscle damage but clearly showed that stress caused the chest problem. Life pressures like this are why your doctor really needs to know your social and occupational situation.

Here's another example. A charming eighty-two-year-old grandmother finally admitted she was having chest pain after three days of discomfort. She called her doctor, who directed her to the emergency room. After three days in the hospital and many tests, the doctors felt she was fine to return home. They increased her heart medication. But it wasn't until her daughter-in-law collared one of the attending physicians in the hospital hallway and asked, "Did she mention that her grandson was getting a divorce and that's been bothering her?" that they put all the pieces together.

The doctors had been busy conducting sophisticated stress tests and medical procedures and had not looked at the whole person. If they had, they would have seen a dear woman whose heart literally ached. When the initial medical history was taken in the ER, she, of course, had not mentioned her family distress. Had the doctor asked or had she thought it relevant, such information would have been a key point in her medical history.

Your family history is also crucial for the doctor to know. We should each have a general understanding of the health of our first-degree relatives and that includes mother, father, aunts and uncles, and of course brothers and sisters. This is especially relevant for heart disease, certain neurologic disorders, allergies and certainly for cancer. [See chapter 8 for more details on how to gather your family history.]

At the end of the medical history taking or at the end of the consultation, you should have a feeling of closure. Have your issues been addressed courteously and professionally?

Your physical examination

This typically follows the taking of the medical history. Up to this point, I hope you have been sitting comfortably either in an exam room chair or in the doctor's personal office having a face-to-face discussion without distractions. With all your clothes on.

In most circumstances, at least for a general medical examination or for your first visit, you will eventually be asked to disrobe completely. You will be asked to wear a paper or cloth gown, which may or may not have sleeves. The doctor's staff will take and note your vital signs. This consists of your pulse, temperature, weight and blood pressure.

Following a washing of the hands as a symbolic way of starting the physical exam, the doctor will listen to your heart and lungs through a stethoscope and will typically feel around your neck, under your arms, breasts, abdomen, the rectum, and carefully examine your skin throughout the whole process. The doctor also may place the stethoscope on your neck to hear your carotid arteries. These main blood vessels supply blood and life-sustaining oxygen to your brain. A blockage here can lead to stroke and death. If there is a characteristic noise in the carotid called a bruit, this might reflect a decreased blood supply (think blockage here), and then your doctor may recommend a more sophisticated test with an ultrasound.

The knees and ankles typically are tapped with a reflex hammer. The doctor will use a lighted instrument to examine your eyes, mouth and ears.

The physical exam should not be painful, but it can be somewhat embarrassing and rather uncomfortable as your abdomen is prodded or your rectum examined. The occurrence of sexually transmitted diseases can be detected by the history and physical examination.

Usually, the history taking would take about ten to fifteen minutes based on the complexity of your case, and the physical exam an equal amount of time. If your doctor has slotted ten minutes for your first exam, you simply won't have enough time for either of you, so make sure when you make your appointment, you have asked for adequate time. Otherwise, you may have to return to continue the history and physical. And that's not fair to you.

TOP TEN SYMPTOMS NOT TO IGNORE (SO DON'T WAIT UNTIL YOUR NEXT PHYSICAL EXAM)

1. **Fatigue** of more than one week's duration without obvious explanation: If you have the flu or are recovering from a surgery or accident, feeling tired is normal. However, hoist the red flags if you're tired for no obvious reason, if you find yourself running out of steam in the early to mid-afternoon, if you push yourself during the week only to collapse in a heap on the weekend, or if you become listless and indifferent to your normal responsibilities. Fatigue usually does not represent a significant problem, but if it lasts more than a week and there are no obvious explanations, see your doctor.

2. **Cough:** We all cough. That is just the nature of the lives we live. A cough that lasts more than five to ten days, especially if you are a smoker and particularly if you start coughing up thick green or ropy phlegm or have blood in your phlegm, is something to be concerned about. And I'm talking about lung cancer. Shortness of breath and weight loss associated with a cough are serious. See your doctor right away.

3. **Pain:** As we get older, we all have aches and pains. Almost always these are not significant. But if persistent pain lasts more than three to five days in a very specific area without obvious explanation, you should have it checked out. Obviously, if you have fallen and hurt your shoulder or banged your knee on the bedpost, you'll have pain. But any pain that comes out of nowhere, that awakens you at night, and clearly does not improve, should be checked.

4. **Chest pain:** Here's the big one many men and women foolishly ignore. Chest pain that occurs if you exert yourself and chest pain that might be described as a squeezing or heavy feeling in your chest could indicate a heart attack. If the pain extends into your jaw or left shoulder, you are toying with disaster. Don't wait for all these symptoms to appear or disappear. Get emergency care now.

(continued on following page)

5. **Blood:** Blood in the rectum, stool, urine or phlegm is a signal. With a vigorous wiping of the rectal/anal area, it is not surprising that the toilet paper might have a pink tinge. Almost never is this a cause for alarm. However, if there is obvious blood on the stool (take a look), and if there is pain with passing a bowel movement, this usually is caused by hemorrhoids. These are prominent blood vessels around the anal opening much like a small group of grapes. Here's the fatal pitfall. It is easy to think the blood from your rectum may be caused by hemorrhoids, when in fact you may have an underlying cancer. That's why, especially in adults, this symptom should not be ignored. If you have a family history of colorectal cancer, all the more reason to see your doctor and check the source of the blood.

6. **A new lump or bump:** This means a lump or bump that is not particularly painful, and one that has not been associated with trauma. Cancer usually is not painful. A lump or bump that has occurred relatively quickly and feels tender is almost always not a cancer. But if it doesn't disappear over a week or so and you can't remember if you hurt yourself there, a professional evaluation would be important.

7. **Moles:** Malignant melanoma is one of the most rapidly increasing cancers. This is also called black-mole cancer and is a virulent group of cancer cells. If a mole rapidly appears, or darkens or itches over a relatively short number of months, or starts to bleed, you need to have a biopsy (cells are then viewed under a microscope).

8. **Weight loss:** As a society, we are consumed with diets. Don't think so? Check out the tabloids as you go through the checkout line in the supermarket. But weight loss without a diet is another matter. Many people who experience a dramatic loss of weight might dance in the street. Some of us pay a lot of money for diet plans to do just that. But a relatively quick loss

(continued on following page)

of weight—faster than two or three pounds a week—may signal an underlying problem such as a thyroid gland that needs to be addressed. Weight loss is commonly a concern if you lose 10 percent of your body weight over a three-month period, yet you haven't changed your eating habits or increased your physical activity.

9. **Headaches:** We all get headaches. We live in a tense society. Headaches often are related to tension and stress and rarely are brain tumors, although that can be your first thought. Don't ignore the relatively new onset of a new type of headache, especially if it occurs in the morning and increases when you cough or sneeze, because that combination could signal a serious condition.

10. **Stroke signs:** Weakness of an arm or a leg or numbness and tingling of an arm, leg, the face or tongue, or difficulty with speech, could indicate the potential onset of a stroke. Stroke causes the death of brain tissue because the blood supply to certain parts of your brain is interrupted. This is an emergency. Don't wait for symptoms to go away, because sometimes these mini-strokes or transient ischemic attacks (TIAs) return in the "big one." And you may not survive that stroke.

I find that many patients cannot be expected to have the sophistication to accurately describe many of these symptoms. Often, our patients might say, "Doc, I just don't feel right. I feel lousy." You cannot know if these are a big deal, a little deal or a minor nuisance. At this point in an office visit, the careful physician, the thoughtful physician, will encourage you to elaborate on how you're feeling and then with insight, professionalism and judgment, the physician can outline the most appropriate tests to hone in on your problem.

As the patient, you should expect that your doctor will not interrupt you. The problem is that many physicians from experience can quickly sense that the complaint or description is not serious, and they interject before the patient has finished speaking. This is not courteous, it is not fair, and it may overlook some underlying and serious problems.

Routine testing

Someone going through an executive health program would have all these routine tests performed:

- **Complete blood count:** The doctor may ask a medical assistant to draw one or two vials of blood from a vein in your arm. This blood is sent to a laboratory, and the results are reported back to the doctor who will discuss the results with you and contact you if there are any concerns. The complete blood count basically looks for evidence of anemia (low red blood cells) and measures the infection-fighting (white blood cells) as well as immune-related cells and those cells related to blood clotting, which are called platelets.

- **Glucose:** This is a test for sugar that is measured using your blood. If you are asked to fast before your blood is drawn at your appointment, don't eat for six to eight hours. Usually, black coffee without cream is allowed, as are unlimited fluids such as water.

- **Blood chemistries:** The blood chemistries—also determined from a sample of your blood—measure the balance of your body minerals as well as how well your liver and kidneys are working. It's amazing what we can tell from blood. These are generic, off-the-shelf screening studies. If any of these measures are abnormal (too high or too low), your doctor will follow up with additional tests.

  Commonly performed blood chemistries measure levels of sodium, potassium, total protein, calcium, liver tests (AST and SGOT), alkaline phosphatase, creatinine and uric acid.

- **Lipid screen** (total cholesterol, HDL, triglycerides, calculated LDL): The lipid screen assesses your total cholesterol—both good and bad types—as well as triglycerides. This is a barometer of fitness and might also indicate the potential role of weight reduction, physical activity or the use of medication. Many people know their total cholesterol level and can have this screened at a shopping center, drugstore or community health fair. But the overall measures of the kinds of cholesterol (both good HDL and bad LDL) along with triglycerides give a better picture of your heart health and potential risk for heart disease.

- **Iron:** If you are having a first-time physical, the doctor may also check your serum iron and iron-binding capacity because this would help screen for disorders of iron metabolism such as hemachromatosis—a condition in which you have too much iron in your blood. This is treatable, but we need to know about it.

- **Other blood tests** may be ordered to look at how well your thyroid is working, to rule out certain sexually transmitted diseases, a blood level for certain medications whose effects are determined by the amount of the substance in your bloodstream, and any number of other measures your doctor may be checking.

- **Urinalysis:** The urinalysis looks for evidence of red blood cells, infection or protein in a sample of your urine. If blood is present in the sample, you may need additional tests. If protein is present to a significant degree, this could indicate kidney disease.

- **Nutrition class:** Usually, if a patient is generally healthy, there is no need for a nutrition class, but if a patient has kidney disease or certain intestinal diseases such as sprue or colitis, there might be a role for consultation with a dietitian.

  Patients usually are asked to fill out a food diary, which outlines what they eat over several typical days. Dietitians are subspecialized much like medical-care providers. In the Mayo Clinic program, our patients may meet with a dietitian for heart disease, renal (kidney) disease, intestinal diseases or specifically focusing on diabetes. Your doctor may refer you to a specialist in your community, or you can locate a qualified dietitian through a medical center. I suggest you work with a registered dietitian—someone with an R.D. degree. Stay away from anyone who professes to be a "nutritionist." You often find less-than-qualified nutrition advisers working in health clubs who want you to buy a host of supplements and vitamins.

- **Chest x-ray:** The chest x-ray makes an image of the size of your heart and allows us to look at the presence or absence of spots in your lungs. Some studies suggest that in the nonsmoker who is generally healthy, the chest x-ray is not a consistently helpful tool, but it generally continues to be ordered.

- **EKG:** This is a tracing of your heart, known as an electrocardiogram or EKG. You see these on TV doctor shows all the time. The patient is hooked up to twelve wires, which are attached in an array across your bare chest. It's not a shock or uncomfortable or painful at all. The EKG measures your heart rhythm and prints out a strip of blips. This test is a general screen for any evidence of heart disease. Doctors can tell from the pattern what may be going on if you have irregular heart rhythms or problems.

- **Vision and hearing screening:** If we have any concerns about vision or hearing, we will have our patients checked by these individual areas. Most doctors don't conduct vision exams like you would have done at a vision center where you might be fitted for eyeglasses. But if you have any medical problems with your eyes, your doctor would refer you to a medical doctor called an ophthalmologist for a further check. Hearing screening, too, is best performed by an audiologist in a soundproof room with very sophisticated equipment. Structural ear problems can be addressed if you are referred to a specialist known as an otorhinolaryngologist.

- **Immunization review and update:** Adults need shots, too, just like children do. Just recently, the Centers for Disease Control and Prevention (CDC) developed a schedule of immunizations for adults. This includes a flu shot every year, especially for those at higher risk, such as the elderly and those with weakened immune systems, and now the flu shot is recommended for everyone over age fifty. And the pneumonia shot is a wise choice. It's just one injection at any age and a revaccination if you're over sixty-five.

  Talk with your doctor about getting protected against hepatitis A and B. People working in medical occupations should be immunized. Tetanus is an every-ten-year thing, so don't wait to step on a nail in your yard or to be snared by a stray fish hook to get a booster. Some adults may even benefit from catching up their childhood vaccinations for measles, mumps, rubella, and now, chicken pox.

  Immunizations are especially important if you travel overseas. The CDC has complete tracking on what shots are needed for certain nasty diseases you'd never be exposed to in the United States, depending on where you're headed. I suggest checking the CDC Web site well in advance of any overseas travel, especially if you're going someplace exotic.

- **Treadmill exercise test and cardiovascular health clinic consultation:** We really do get physical and put our patients through a treadmill test when we first see them and every five years after that. We tape electrodes for an EKG, the heart tracing, on the chest and put our patients on a treadmill to begin brisk walking. Usually, fatigue signals the end of the test, or we stop the testing if we see abnormalities on the cardiogram.

- **Thyroid-stimulating hormone (TSH):** The thyroid-stimulating hormone is measured in blood, or should be checked yearly at age forty and older. High or low levels indicate the health of your thyroid gland. Thyroid conditions can be treated, but we need to monitor these hormone levels carefully.
- **Vitamin B$_{12}$:** We also measure vitamin B$_{12}$ levels to pinpoint a difficult-to-detect disease called pernicious anemia—a condition that shows up in older people. This is easily treated with vitamin B$_{12}$ injections or an oral form of the medication.
- **Colon:** The gold standard for detection of cancer of the colon remains a colonoscopy. Usually this is started at about age forty or fifty, and repeated every five years or so based on your risk.
- **Bone density:** The role of assessing for the bone-thinning condition known as osteoporosis remains controversial. Most clinicians would recommend a bone density assessment at about the time of menopause for women or earlier if there is a strong positive family history or disorders that might be associated with osteoporosis such as for heavy smokers and women who are relatively inactive. We also test bone density in men. The test is a simple x-ray of your hip and spine taken while you lie on an x-ray table with your legs elevated on a foam block. Simple. The quick tests done at health fairs and shopping center screenings, in which bone density is measured through your wrist, finger or heel, are just mass screening devices for awareness. If you try one of these tests and you are judged to have low bone density, get the full spine and hip screening before you and your doctor make any decisions about treatment.
- **Prostate specific antigen (PSA):** For men, most medical authorities recommend an early PSA starting at age fifty, but in the African American community—especially if there is a strong family history of cancer of the prostate—the PSA typically is started much earlier, even at age forty.
- **Mammogram:** Most medical groups recommend mammograms starting at age forty to be given every year.
- **Pap smear:** A Pap smear usually is performed every one to three years but more frequently in sexually active women or someone who has multiple sexual partners.
- **Mental health:** Most clinicians do not routinely screen for depression unless there are some clear-cut indications that this is of concern. Patients usually don't come in and announce they are depressed,

although we are encouraged by campaigns to raise awareness about this highly treatable condition. But if a patient talks about not sleeping, not eating, gaining a lot of weight, or the joy in life just not being there, we can ask leading questions to get to the heart of the matter.

Obviously, the general medical exam needs to be focused on your specific needs, but this is the battery of testing we follow for our patients. Any test or examination by your doctor needs to be carefully interpreted for you, especially laboratory tests that take a few days for results to come back.

I don't think it's enough for you to receive a postcard in the mail with boxes checked that say "normal." If you're comfortable with that, fine. But I advise you to discuss your test results by phone with the doctor or in person. That way your questions can be answered on the spot. Tell the doctor you expect to hear from him or her by phone. And continue to follow up with the doctor's office until you get an answer.

Also don't be comforted if the doctor's office says, "We'll call you if you have any abnormal results." You could easily slip through the cracks in a poorly designed alert system like that. Don't settle for a no-news-is-good-news plan. You want to hear the news, whatever it is, even if you have to keep calling the office. **Do it.**

Many patients are asking for lab results to be faxed to them, and if you want copies, set this up before you leave the office. That way you can start building your own medical record file. Or ask the office to mail you a copy. If they require a release form, sign that before you leave as well.

My Thoughts . . .

Screening is a mantra embedded into the fabric of the American Cancer Society. The earlier a cancer is detected and treated, the better the prognosis. **I know of no cancer in which the prognosis of a far-advanced cancer is better than that of an early-stage cancer.** Therefore, individuals and their health-care providers should be in a partnership to outline acceptable screening studies to detect cancer in a curable stage.

One of the greatest deterrents and one of the strongest arsenals against disease is having a relationship with a primary health-care professional who can provide access to the medical system and can appropriately interpret signs and symptoms. Equally important, careful physical examination and a thorough medical history may detect an early-stage illness or developing condition when it is potentially curable and probably controllable.

Use the health partnership you have created with your doctor, nurse practitioner or physician's assistant. This is the person you can talk to and in whom you trust. But ultimately your health is in your hands. No one has a greater stake in your health than you do.

We are each on a journey. An overarching theme of life is to have meaning and purpose. Without that, there is no reason to go on. "Give me a reason to live, and I will find a way to live," wrote Viktor Frankl in *Man's Search for Meaning*.

We each have the possibilities, gifts and talents to remake the world in some small way. But we cannot do that without health—the greatest of all blessings. Give a man a fish and he will no longer go hungry, but teach him how to fish, and he then learns to feed his soul. In a way, I hope you are learning how to fish . . . not for trout but for well-being.

So what is this all about? Unless we take personal responsibility for our own health and welfare and unless we recognize that we, indeed, can do something about our health, we may well be bitterly disappointed. As Walt Whitman said, we are captains of our souls, and we need to be appropriately active and assertive in caring for our own health and wellness. After all, he who has health has everything. He who does not have health has nothing.

But sometimes, despite all the healthful eating and exercise and "good living," we lose our health, and the journey to regain it can often take us down paths we never wanted to travel. Not only cancer takes us on a new uncharted path, but any dread disease or chronic condition can turn our lives around completely.

Few diseases rival cancer for an emotional blow, but we need to acknowledge that other dreadful diseases can cut us down just when we think we are on top of our game. Illness does not respect status, fame or your checkbook. Focus on the coping skills and navigational tools to weather the cancer storm, but the tactics and strategies are similar regardless of your disease. If we are lost in the woods, the way to survive is the same whether we're lost in a national park in California or the Everglades in Florida.

Starting with the next chapter, I have drawn up your survival map.

> The following worksheets from the American Cancer Society summarize all the tests and procedures explained in this chapter. Please use these worksheets to develop your own action plan for early detection and discuss these with your doctor.

Cancer Prevention and Early Detection Worksheet for Men

While a tremendous amount of progress has been made in cancer research, we still don't understand exactly what causes most cancers. However, we do know of many factors that place us at increased risk for different cancers. Some of these factors are beyond our control, but there are others that we can do something about. And today, more than ever before, we have screening tests available to help us detect some cancers in their earliest stages.

Below you will find helpful information on the most common cancers that can affect you as a man—what puts you at risk, how you can lower this risk, and ways that you can make sure that if you do develop cancer, it is found early, when it is most easily treated. The final column on the worksheet allows room for you to write down your own plan of action to combat cancer.

It's important to realize that some factors may place you at higher risk than others, and some behaviors may lower your risk more than others. Many cancers develop without any of these risk factors present. There is not enough room here to go into more detail—this is intended only as a general guide. For a more thorough explanation of cancer risk factors, visit our Cancer Resource Center at *www.cancer.org*, or call us any time, day or night, at 1-800-ACS-2345. And if you have any risk factors or haven't had your early detection tests, please take this worksheet and discuss this with your doctor.

Screening for Cancer in General

The American Cancer Society recommends that all men get a cancer-related checkup every 3 years between the ages of 20 and 40, and every year thereafter. This checkup should include health counseling and, depending on a person's age, might include examinations for cancers of the skin, thyroid, mouth, lymph nodes and testes, as well as for some diseases other than cancer.

Special tests for certain cancers are recommended as outlined below.

Reprinted by the permission of the American Cancer Society, Inc. We're available to answer your questions about cancer any time, day or night. Call us at 1-800-ACS-2345, or visit us online at *www.cancer.org*.

Prostate Cancer

Risk Factors	Preventive Behaviors	Screening Tests	Your Action Plan:
• Are you over age 50? • Are you African American? • Do you eat a diet high in fat? • Are you overweight? • Are you inactive? • Do you have a family history of prostate cancer?	• Eating a diet low in fat and high in vegetables, fruits, and grains. • Getting at least 30 minutes of physical activity on most days. • Achieving and maintaining a healthy weight.	• Consider a yearly PSA blood test and digital rectal exam starting at age 50, or at age 45 if you are at high risk (African American, or have a father or brother diagnosed with prostate cancer at a young age). • Talk to your doctor about the pros and cons of prostate cancer screening.	Steps to Lower Your Risk: Screening:

Lung Cancer

Risk Factors	Preventive Behaviors	Screening Tests	Your Action Plan:
• Do you smoke tobacco? • Do you work around asbestos? • Have you been exposed to radon? • Have you been exposed to uranium? • Have you been exposed to arsenic? • Have you been exposed to vinyl chloride? • Do you smoke marijuana? • Are you regularly exposed to secondhand smoke?	• Quitting smoking. • Encouraging those you live with or work with to quit. • If you smoke, let your doctor know if you develop any of the following symptoms (some may have causes other than cancer): • A cough that does not go away • Chest pain, often aggravated by deep breathing • Hoarseness • Weight loss and loss of appetite • Bloody or rust-colored sputum (spit or phlegm) • Shortness of breath • Fever without a known reason • Recurring infections such as bronchitis and pneumonia • New onset of wheezing	None have been found to be effective. Usually found on x-ray, but there are often no symptoms. • Talk to your doctor about possible screening if you have any of the risk factors listed.	Steps to Lower Your Risk: Screening:

Reprinted by the permission of the American Cancer Society, Inc. We're available to answer your questions about cancer any time, day or night. Call us at 1-800-ACS-2345, or visit us online at www.cancer.org.

Colorectal Cancer

Risk Factors	Preventive Behaviors	Screening Tests	Your Action Plan:
• Do you have a family history of colon or rectal cancer? • Do you have a colorectal cancer syndrome in your family (such as familial adenomatous polyposis (FAP) or hereditary nonpolyposis colon cancer (HNPCC))? • Do you have a personal history of colorectal cancer? • Do you have a personal history of intestinal polyps? • Do you have a personal history of chronic inflammatory bowel disease (Crohn's disease or ulcerative colitis)? • Are you over 50 years of age? • Do you consume a diet mostly from animal sources? • Are you physically inactive? • Are you overweight? • Do you use tobacco?	• Following screening guidelines to remove adenomatous polyps before they become cancer. • Getting at least 30 minutes of physical activity on most days. • Achieving and maintaining a healthy weight. Eating plenty of fruits, vegetables, and whole grain foods and limiting intake of high-fat foods. • Quitting smoking.	**Beginning at age 50, you should follow one of the five screening options below:** • Yearly fecal occult blood test (FOBT) • Flexible sigmoidoscopy every 5 years • Yearly fecal occult blood test plus flexible sigmoidoscopy every 5 years *(Of the options above, the American Cancer Society prefers yearly FOBT combined with flexible sigmoidoscopy every 5 years)* • Double-contrast barium enema every 5 years • Colonoscopy every 10 years Talk to your doctor about beginning screening earlier and/or more often if you have any of the following risk factors: • Strong family history of colorectal cancer or polyps (cancer or polyps in a first-degree relative younger than 60 or in two first-degree relatives of any age). Note: a first-degree relative is defined as a parent, sibling, or child. • A known family history of colorectal cancer syndromes • A personal history of colorectal cancer or adenomatous polyps • A personal history of chronic inflammatory bowel disease	Steps to Lower Your Risk: Screening:

Skin Cancer

Risk Factors	Preventive Behaviors	Screening Tests	Your Action Plan:

• Do you sunbathe?
• Do you use tanning booths?
• Do you have fair skin with blonde or red hair?
• Do you sunburn easily or have many freckles?
• Did you have severe sunburns as a child?
• Do you have many or unusually shaped moles?
• Do you live in a southern climate or at a high altitude?
• Do you spend a lot of time outdoors (for work or recreation)?
• Have you ever received radiation treatments?
• Do you have a family history of skin cancer?
• Do you have a weakened immune system due to an organ transplant or due to another condition?
• Were you born with xeroderma pigmentosum (XP), basal cell nevus syndrome, or dysplastic nevus syndrome?
• Have you been exposed to any of the following chemicals?
  • Arsenic
  • Coal tar
  • Paraffin
  • Radium
	• Staying out of the sun, especially between 10 A.M. and 4 P.M.
	• Wearing a broad-brimmed hat, a shirt, and sunglasses when out in the sun.
	• Using a sunscreen with an SPF of 15 or higher, and reapplying it often.
	• Not using tanning beds or sunlamps.
	• Protecting young children from excess sun exposure.
	• Checking your skin regularly for abnormal or changing areas, especially moles, and having them examined by your doctor.
		Cancer-Related Checkup (including skin exam):
		
		• **Over 20:** every 3 years
		• **Over 40:** every year
		
		Self-exam (monthly):
		
		• Become familiar with any moles, freckles or other abnormalities on your skin. Use a mirror or have a family member or close friend look at areas you can't see (ears, scalp, lower back).
		• Check for changes once a month. Show any suspicious or changing areas to your doctor.
			Steps to Lower Your Risk:
			
			Screening:

Reprinted by the permission of the American Cancer Society, Inc. We're available to answer your questions about cancer any time, day or night. Call us at 1-800-ACS-2345, or visit us online at *www.cancer.org*.

Cancer Prevention and Early Detection Worksheet for Women

While a tremendous amount of progress has been made in cancer research, we still don't understand exactly what causes most cancers. However, we know of many factors that place us at increased risk for different cancers. Some of these factors are beyond our control, but there are others that we can do something about. And today, more than ever before, we have screening tests available to help us detect some cancers in their earliest stages.

Below you will find helpful information on the most common cancers that can affect you as a woman—what puts you at risk, how you can lower this risk, and ways that you can make sure that if you do develop cancer, it is found early, when it is most easily treated. The final column on each sheet allows room for you to develop your own plan of action to combat cancer.

It's important to realize that some factors may place you at higher risk than others, and some behaviors may lower your risk more than others. Many cancers develop without any of these risk factors present. There is not enough room here to go into more detail—this is intended only as a general guide. For a more thorough explanation of cancer risk factors, visit our Cancer Resource Center at *www.cancer.org*, or call us any time, day or night, at 1-800-ACS-2345. And if you have any risk factors or haven't had your early detection tests, please take this worksheet and discuss this with your doctor.

Screening for Cancer in General

The American Cancer Society recommends that all women get a cancer-related checkup every 3 years between the ages of 20 and 40, and every year thereafter. This checkup should include health counseling and, depending on a person's age, might include examinations for cancers of the skin, thyroid, mouth, lymph nodes, and ovaries, as well as for some diseases other than cancer.

Special tests for certain cancers are recommended as outlined below.

Reprinted by the permission of the American Cancer Society, Inc. We're available to answer your questions about cancer any time, day or night. Call us at 1-800-ACS-2345, or visit us online at *www.cancer.org*.

Lung Cancer

Risk Factors	Preventive Behaviors	Screening Tests	Your Action Plan:

• Do you smoke tobacco?
• Do you work around asbestos?
• Have you been exposed to radon?
• Have you been exposed to uranium?
• Have you been exposed to arsenic?
• Have you been exposed to vinyl chloride?
• Do you smoke marijuana?
• Are you regularly exposed to secondhand smoke?
	• Quitting smoking.
	• Encouraging those you live with or work with to quit.
	• If you smoke, let your doctor know if you develop any of the following symptoms (some may have causes other than cancer):
	  • A cough that does not go away
	  • Chest pain, often aggravated by deep breathing
	  • Hoarseness
	  • Weight loss and loss of appetite
	  • Bloody or rust-colored sputum (spit or phlegm)
	  • Shortness of breath
	  • Fever without a known reason
	  • Recurring infections such as bronchitis and pneumonia
	  • New onset of wheezing
		None have been found effective. Usually found on x-ray, but there are often no symptoms.
		
		• Talk to your doctor about possible screening if you have any of the risk factors listed.
			Steps to Lower Your Risk:
			
			Screening:

Reprinted by the permission of the American Cancer Society, Inc. We're available to answer your questions about cancer any time, day or night. Call us at 1-800-ACS-2345, or visit us online at *www.cancer.org.*

Colorectal Cancer

Risk Factors	Preventive Behaviors	Screening Tests	Your Action Plan:
• Do you have a family history of colon or rectal cancer? • Do you have a colorectal cancer syndrome in your family (such as familial adenomatous polyposis (FAP) or hereditary nonpolyposis colon cancer (HNPCC))? • Do you have a personal history of colorectal cancer? • Do you have a personal history of intestinal polyps? • Do you have a personal history of chronic inflammatory bowel disease (Crohn's disease or ulcerative colitis)? • Are you over 50 years of age? • Do you consume a diet mostly from animal sources? • Are you physically inactive? • Are you overweight? • Do you use tobacco?	• Following screening guidelines to remove adenomatous polyps before they become cancer • Getting at least 30 minutes of physical activity on most days • Achieving and maintaining a healthy weight • Eating plenty of fruits, vegetables, and whole grain foods, and limiting intake of high-fat foods • Quitting smoking	**Beginning at age 50, you should follow *one* of the five screening options below:** • Yearly fecal occult blood test (FOBT) • Flexible sigmoidoscopy every 5 years • Yearly fecal occult blood test plus flexible sigmoidoscopy every 5 years *(Of the options above, the American Cancer Society prefers yearly FOBT combined with flexible sigmoidoscopy every 5 years)* • Double-contrast barium enema every 5 years • Colonoscopy every 10 years Talk to your doctor about beginning screening earlier and/or more often if you have any of the following risk factors: • Strong family history of colorectal cancer or polyps (cancer or polyps in a first-degree relative younger than 60 or in two first-degree relatives of any age). Note: a first-degree relative is defined as a parent, sibling, or child. • A known family history of colorectal cancer syndromes • A personal history of colorectal cancer or adenomatous polyps • A personal history of chronic inflammatory bowel disease	Steps to Lower Your Risk: Screening:

Reprinted by the permission of the American Cancer Society, Inc. We're available to answer your questions about cancer any time, day or night. Call us at 1-800-ACS-2345, or visit us online at *www.cancer.org*.

Skin Cancer

Risk Factors	Preventive Behaviors	Screening Tests	Your Action Plan:

• Do you sunbathe?
• Do you use tanning booths?
• Do you have fair skin with blonde or red hair?
• Do you sunburn easily or have many freckles?
• Did you have severe sunburns as a child?
• Do you have many or unusually shaped moles?
• Do you live in a southern climate or at a high altitude?
• Do you spend a lot of time outdoors (for work or recreation)?
• Have you ever received radiation treatments?
• Do you have a family history of skin cancer?
• Do you have a weakened immune system due to an organ transplant or due to another condition?
• Were you born with xeroderma pigmentosum (XP), basal cell nevus syndrome, or dysplastic nevus syndrome?
• Have you been exposed to any of the following chemicals?
  • Arsenic
  • Coal tar
  • Paraffin
  • Radium
	• Staying out of the sun, especially between 10 A.M. and 4 P.M.
	• Wearing a broad-brimmed hat, a shirt, and sunglasses when out in the sun.
	• Using a sunscreen with an SPF of 15 or higher, and reapplying it often.
	• Not using tanning beds or sunlamps.
	• Protecting young children from excess sun exposure.
	• Checking your skin regularly for abnormal or changing areas, especially moles, and having them examined by your doctor.
		Cancer-Related Checkup (including skin exam):
		• **Over 20:** every 3 years
		• **Over 40:** every year
		
		Self-exam (monthly):
		• Become familiar with any moles, freckles or other abnormalities on your skin. Use a mirror or have a family member or close friend look at areas you can't see (ears, scalp, lower back).
		• Check for changes once a month. Show any suspicious or changing areas to your doctor.
			Steps to Lower Your Risk:
			
			Screening:

Reprinted by the permission of the American Cancer Society, Inc. We're available to answer your questions about cancer any time, day or night. Call us at 1-800-ACS-2345, or visit us online at *www.cancer.org*.

Cervical Cancer

Risk Factors	Preventive Behaviors	Screening Tests	Your Action Plan:

• Were you (are you) sexually active before age 17?
 • Have you had multiple sex partners or a partner who has had multiple partners?
 • Have you had unprotected sex?
 • Do you have a history of a sexually transmitted disease (especially HPV with genital warts), or HIV?
 • Do you smoke?
 • Do you eat a diet low in fruits and vegetables?
 • Did your mother take diethylstilbestrol (DES) during her pregnancy?
 • Are you over age 50?
	• Abstaining from or practicing safer sex using barrier protection each time you have intercourse
	 • Quitting smoking
	 • Eating a diet rich in fruits and vegetables
	 • Watching for and reporting signs and symptoms (although all of these can have other causes):
	   • Abnormal uterine bleeding or spotting
	   • Abnormal vaginal discharge
	   • Pain during intercourse
		• Yearly pelvic exam with Pap test to begin at age 18 or when sexually active, whichever is earlier
		 • After three or more consecutive satisfactory normal yearly examinations, the Pap test may be performed less frequently at the discretion of your doctor
			Steps to Lower Your Risk:
			
			 Screening:

Reprinted by the permission of the American Cancer Society, Inc. We're available to answer your questions about cancer any time, day or night. Call us at 1-800-ACS-2345, or visit us online at *www.cancer.org*.

Breast Cancer

Risk Factors	Preventive Behaviors	Screening Tests	Your Action Plan:
• Are you over age 50? • Do you have a personal history of breast cancer? • Do you have a family history of breast cancer (especially mother, sister, or daughter)? • Did you have your first child after age 30 (or have no children)? • Did you have chest radiation as a child or young woman as treatment for another cancer? • Did you begin menstruating before age 12, or go through menopause after age 50? • Have you been on hormone replacement therapy for more than 5 years? • Do you drink one or more alcoholic beverages a day? • Are you physically inactive? • If you are postmenopausal, have you gained weight, especially around your waist?	• Following recommended guidelines for early detection of breast cancer • Talking with your doctor about the risks and benefits of hormone replacement therapy for your risk of cancer and other diseases (like heart disease and osteoporosis) • Getting at least 30 minutes of physical activity on most days • Achieving and maintaining a healthy weight • Eating plenty of fruits, vegetables, and whole grain foods and limiting intake of high-fat foods • Decreasing your alcohol intake **Women at high risk:** • Considering taking tamoxifen or enrolling in a chemoprevention study (for more information, see our document "Tamoxifen and Raloxifene: Questions & Answers") • Talking with your doctor about more frequent tests for early detection	**Age 20–39:** • Breast self examination each month • Clinical breast examination by health care professional every three years **Age 40 and over:** • Yearly mammogram • Yearly clinical breast examination by a health care professional, near the time of the mammogram • Breast self-exam every month	Steps to Lower Your Risk: Screening:

Reprinted by the permission of the American Cancer Society, Inc. We're available to answer your questions about cancer any time, day or night. Call us at 1-800-ACS-2345, or visit us online at www.cancer.org.

Endometrial Cancer

Risk Factors	Preventive Behaviors	Screening Tests	Your Action Plan:
• Are you over age 40? • Did you begin menstruating before age 12, or go through menopause after age 50? • Do you have a history of infertility or never giving birth? • Are you obese (very overweight)? • Do you eat a diet high in animal fat? • Do you have a history of diabetes? • Have you taken tamoxifen or long-term estrogen replacement therapy without progesterone (if you still have your uterus)? • Do you have a history of breast or ovarian cancer? • Have you had radiation therapy to your pelvis? • Do you have a family history of hereditary nonpolyposis colorectal cancer (HNPCC), or are you at risk for this cancer?	• Watching for and reporting any abnormal uterine spotting or bleeding • Using oral contraceptives for many years • Talking with your doctor about the risks and benefits of hormone replacement therapy for your risk of cancer and other diseases (like heart disease and osteoporosis) • If taking hormone replacement therapy with your uterus still intact, taking estrogen with *progesterone*	**Average Risk** • Talk with your doctor, especially at the time of menopause, about the risks and symptoms of endometrial cancer • Report any vaginal bleeding or spotting to your doctor • Yearly pelvic exam **Increased Risk** (includes women with any of the first 9 risk factors in the left column) • Discuss endometrial cancer early detection testing with your doctor. **HNPCC** • If you have or are at risk for HNPCC, consider yearly testing with endometrial biopsy beginning at age 35.	Steps to Lower Your Risk: Screening:

Reprinted by the permission of the American Cancer Society, Inc. We're available to answer your questions about cancer any time, day or night. Call us at 1-800-ACS-2345, or visit us online at *www.cancer.org*.

Ovarian Cancer

Risk Factors	Preventive Behaviors	Screening Tests	Your Action Plan:

• Have you already gone through menopause?
• Did you begin menstruating before age 12, or go through menopause after age 50?
• Did you have your first child after age 30 (or have no children)?
• Do you have a family history of ovarian cancer?
• Do you have a personal history of breast cancer?
• Have you been on hormone replacement therapy for more than 5 years?
	• Using oral contraceptives for several years
	• Watching for and reporting signs and symptoms (although all of these can have other causes):
	  • Abdominal swelling
	  • Vaginal bleeding
	  • Back and/or leg pain
	  • Chronic stomach pain
	• Talking with your doctor about the risks and benefits of hormone replacement therapy and your risks of cancer and other diseases, like heart disease and osteoporosis
	• Talking with your doctor about having your ovaries removed, if you are at high risk. (This surgery causes sudden menopause.)
		There are no effective and proven tests for early detection of ovarian cancer.
		• As part of your regular health maintenance, you should undergo a periodic and thorough pelvic examination as directed by your doctor.
			Steps to Lower Your Risk:
			
			Screening:

Reprinted by the permission of the American Cancer Society, Inc. We're available to answer your questions about cancer any time, day or night. Call us at 1-800-ACS-2345, or visit us online at *www.cancer.org*.

Part Two

WHAT YOUR DOCTOR NEVER TELLS YOU

READER/CUSTOMER CARE SURVEY

We care about your opinions. Please take a moment to fill out this Reader Survey card and mail it back to us.
As a special **"thank you"** we'll send you exciting news about interesting books and a valuable **Gift Certificate.**

Please PRINT using ALL CAPS

First Name [   ] MI. [ ] Last Name [   ]

Address [   ]

City [   ] ST [ ] Zip [   ] — [   ]

Phone # ([   ]) [   ] — [   ]   Fax # ([   ]) [   ] — [   ]

Email [   ]

(1) Gender:
___ Female   ___ Male

(2) Age:
___ 12 or under
___ 13-19
___ 20-39
___ 40-59
___ 60+

(3) Marital Status
___ Married
___ Single
___ Divorced/Widowed

(4) Did you receive this book as a gift?
___ Yes   ___ No

(5) How many Health Communications books have you bought or read?
___ 1   ___ 2-4   ___ 5+

(6) How did you find out about this book?
Please fill in ONE.
1) ___ Recommendation
2) ___ Store Display
3) ___ Bestseller List
4) ___ Online
5) ___ Advertisement
6) ___ Catalog/Mailing
7) ___ Interview/Review (TV, Radio, Print)

(7) Where do you usually buy books?
Please fill in your top TWO choices.
1) ___ Bookstore
2) ___ Religious Bookstore
3) ___ Online
4) ___ Book Club/Mail Order
5) ___ Price Club (Costco, Sam's Club, etc.)
6) ___ Retail Store (Target, Wal-Mart, etc.)

(9) What subjects do you enjoy reading about most? Rank only **FIVE.** Use 1 for your favorite, 2 for second favorite, etc.

	1	2	3	4	5
1) Parenting/Family	○	○	○	○	○
2) Relationships	○	○	○	○	○
3) Recovery/Addictions	○	○	○	○	○
4) Health/Nutrition	○	○	○	○	○
5) Christianity	○	○	○	○	○
6) Spirituality/Inspiration	○	○	○	○	○
7) Business Self-Help	○	○	○	○	○
8) Teen Issues	○	○	○	○	○
9) Sports	○	○	○	○	○

(14) What attracts you most to a book?
(Please rank 1-4 in order of preference.)

	1	2	3	4
1) Title	○	○	○	○
2) Cover Design	○	○	○	○
3) Author	○	○	○	○
4) Content	○	○	○	○

TAPE IN MIDDLE; DO NOT STAPLE

BUSINESS REPLY MAIL
FIRST-CLASS MAIL PERMIT NO 45 DEERFIELD BEACH, FL

POSTAGE WILL BE PAID BY ADDRESSEE

HEALTH COMMUNICATIONS, INC.
3201 SW 15TH STREET
DEERFIELD BEACH FL 33442-9875

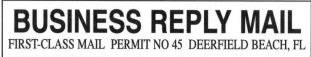

FOLD HERE

Comments:

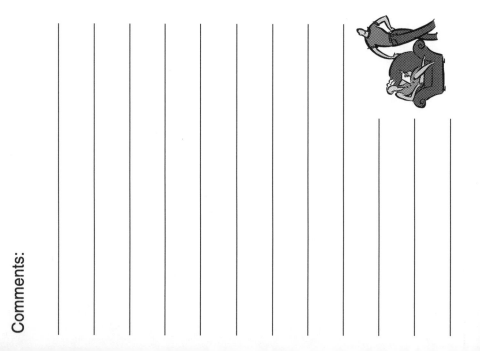

How to Talk So
Your Doctor Will Listen

Never go to a doctor whose office plants have died.

—Erma Bombeck

What's the one question your doctor should always ask you, but rarely ever does?

If your doctor spends time with you, talking about your health, consider yourself very lucky. Some good clinicians can hone in on your major health concerns in just a few minutes. But you need to talk to your doctor, face to face, with your clothes on—and your doctor needs to listen. Here's why.

In conducting a thorough head-to-toe exam, your doctor should start first by asking you this key question: **How are you feeling?** Take that question very seriously. The doctor is looking for any change in your state of good health and really wants to know. Always mention the big things such as weight gain or loss, headaches in the morning or if they awaken you from sleep, difficulty swallowing, shortness of breath and the like. Your doctor should ask you if you have abdominal pain, problems with urination (can't go, go all the time), about lumps and bumps, a sore that doesn't heal, a chronic cough.

If you're a new patient, many doctors ask you to fill out a comprehensive questionnaire that contains a wide range of questions—often as you wait in the waiting room. If your doctor doesn't run through the checklist—head to toe—with you during your regular physical exam, insist on filling this out every time anyway. It just might uncover some health issues you need to bring up during your exam.

If right now you're thinking that your doctor doesn't ask you any questions like this, then maybe you need to find a doctor who does—or work with the doctor you see now by becoming an empowered, proactive patient. Let's look at what you should expect from your doctor and how you can make that encounter more productive.

Why People Don't Go to the Doctor and Why They Should

I'm assuming, of course, that you make regular appointments for the screening tests discussed in the last chapter. We all know about the ninety-year-old lady who seems to be the picture of health and has never been to a doctor "in her life"—or at least since her children were born decades earlier, and even then she didn't need him (yes, they were all men when she was a young woman).

Other people, mostly men, feel it's a sign of weakness to go to a doctor, so men avoid doctors like the plague, even if they thought they had the plague. The prevalence of walk-in, no-waiting clinics has made time in front of an M.D. a little easier and faster, but Americans still practice procrastination when it comes to facing anything medical. It's no mystery why people don't go to the doctor. These excuses may sound familiar:

- I'm too busy.
- I'm okay. I know what's going on. I read about it on the Internet.
- I tried home care, and it seems to be working.
- I don't want the doctor to tell me to stop smoking and drinking.
- The doctor can't help me.
- I'm afraid of needles.
- I don't want to wait.
- I can't afford it. It's not covered by my insurance.
- I don't want to know.
- I don't have a doctor.

And of course there's the old familiar, "I didn't think my symptoms were bad enough." A group of patients were interviewed for a study published in the *British Medical Journal.* Many felt their symptoms weren't severe enough to seek medical care, though all these people were eventually diagnosed with heart attacks! They had been confused about whether they were having chest pain or indigestion, and they had hoped their discomfort would go away. If the symptoms appeared on weekends or at night, these heart attack patients said they were especially reluctant to seek help during these off-hours.

So if people are not seeking medical attention for critical life-threatening conditions like heart attacks, they certainly are not scheduling regular appointments for basic medical screening, and they will continue to find excuses not to.

I recently read about a large managed-care group, and I won't mention the name, that gave bonuses to the telephone-service representatives in their call centers if they reduced the time they spent talking with patients who were calling to schedule doctors' appointments. In addition, the phone reps were financially rewarded if they kept the number of callers actually scheduling appointments between 15 and 35 percent.

Frankly, I had to read the article twice because I simply could not believe that a medical organization was rushing people through the appointment process and, on top of that, discouraging their clients from seeing a doctor. We know it's sometimes quite difficult to pick up the phone and make that call in the first place. We surely don't need more barriers standing between you and medical care.

Happily, however, the medical group dropped the practice. The phone reps, who are not trained health professionals, were being asked to evaluate callers' medical conditions when making appointments or refer them to a nurse advice line, and state law limited those tasks to medical personnel only.

My message to you is this

You don't have to give your medical history or even discuss why you wish to see the doctor with the person who answers the phone at the doctor's office. Your goal is to make an appointment. That's it. Don't let them discourage you from coming in. And if your need is urgent, say so, they'll work you in. If you are not satisfied, ask to speak to the doctor's nurse, who can talk with you immediately and make an assessment or phone you back within a matter of a few hours. They do this all the time. It's part of their job as ringmaster of the doctor's schedule. Generally, the person answering the phone is a scheduler, not a medically trained staff member. Make your wishes known or ask to speak with a higher-level staff member.

Get Your Seven Minutes' Worth

The average doctor visit ranges from just seven to sixteen minutes. Sometimes twenty. You can make those precious minutes productive, or you can sit there and waste "your" time while the doctor never gets around to the "real" reason you showed up in the office. It's proven that many patients (mostly men) finally get around to mentioning the blood in the stool or chest pain when the doctor has his or her hand on the exam room doorknob and is about to exit.

To get your seven minutes' worth, try to be the first patient in the morning. The doctor is fresher and might be more on schedule than later in the day. Chances are you'll get more of the doctor's time. You don't want to be scheduled at 11:30 just before lunch. You're definitely not going to get in on time. Another option is to be the first appointment after lunch. Frankly, the best time for a physical exam is the day after Thanksgiving and the week after Christmas. Most people are not focused on their health, and the waiting rooms are nearly empty.

Bring with you everything you think the doctor may need. In fact, send medical records ahead, especially if you're seeing a new doctor. And I'll discuss medical records in much more detail later in this chapter because they really are vital—you need to keep your own records.

What are your expectations when you visit the doctor? One study in the United Kingdom asked patients in the waiting room what they wanted from their visit to a general practitioner. After the appointment, the researchers asked whether the patients' expectations were met. Most patients wanted the doctor to listen to them and then talk about their concerns. They felt this partnership would result in a mutual agreement about treatment. Patients also wanted the doctors to discuss how to stay healthy and reduce their risks for illness.

Interestingly, in this study, when doctors took the time to have a dialogue about a condition, the patients didn't want (or need) prescription medication. How quickly some doctors dash off a prescription, tear it off the pad, and send the patient packing to the pharmacy, when in fact most patients don't want a prescription at all—a prescription for a healthier life, perhaps, but not necessarily drugs.

Unsaid but not forgotten

"Silence is not always golden," according to University of California-Davis researchers in the *Archives of Internal Medicine,* and what is left unsaid in the exam room is not necessarily forgotten by the patient. This research found that 9 percent of patients had something they wanted to ask their physicians but did not. Subsequently, they reported less improvement in their symptoms. Patients wanted to ask for more medical information, for a physical exam, for a diagnostic test or procedure, new medications, or referral to a specialist—but didn't ask.

Whose fault is that?

Whether the patient felt intimidated or simply forgot, there is a way to assure that your questions will be addressed. I suggest you mail, fax or e-mail your doctor a brief note a day or two ahead of your scheduled appointment to alert the doctor about the major things you are concerned about. Say this: *Dear Dr. Jones, I am looking forward to our appointment on Tuesday. I'm especially concerned about a nagging cough and some pain in my abdomen.* This clues the doctor in to what is going on.

Contrary to what many people do, I advise you *not* to bring a long laundry list of health concerns because you'll get sidetracked on how much calcium you need to take and not get to the much more important concern about morning headaches. But do bring a list of all medications you are taking, their dosages and frequency, and include herbals and vitamins you buy for yourself without a prescription.

Good communication helps you build trust with your doctor and with other caregivers. A study in the *Journal of General Internal Medicine* revealed that up to 12 percent of patients surveyed considered changing doctors who did not inform them of their medical options, who did not offer understandable explanations, who did not take time to answer questions or involve the patient in medical decisions. Only 12 percent? I don't understand why someone would continue to see the same doctor who engendered distrust. You don't have to.

I asked [my doctors] if I'd be able to play singles tennis, and they said I could. That made me very happy since I haven't played in five years.

—Walter Cronkite

Who teaches doctors to listen?

Actually, no one teaches doctors to listen. Not in medical school. Medical students and residents receive little effective training in the human interactions of their craft, according to a consensus of expert teachers reported in *The Journal of the American Medical Association*. Humanism in medicine can be taught only at the bedside. That's where I have polished my skills, and I teach others in my role as professor at the Mayo Medical School.

Some medical schools teach interviewing skills. Our students role-play with each other and with medical-school faculty. Valuable skills are taught, such as introducing yourself to the patient and making eye contact. We want our doctors to use language patients can understand. It's one thing to dictate a diagnosis of hypercholesterolemia for the patient's chart, but that means nothing to the patient until the doctor explains it means high cholesterol. And then takes it further by explaining what cholesterol is and how it affects the heart and risk for heart attack. If your doctor uses terms you don't understand, by all means, stop and ask, "What are you saying?" or "Can you help me understand what that means to me?"

We in the medical-school faculty are trying to convey to our students that the doctor–patient relationship should be a partnership. The paternalistic Marcus Welby, M.D., who made housecalls, is a thing of the past.

We see our patients in tiny exam rooms and offices. This is an environment where patients are not always comfortable. Granted we are not all excellent communicators, but this face-to-face encounter clearly is an interaction that we can teach our medical students to handle well. Many medical schools now have video-tapings of experienced clinicians evaluating patients and also residents, interns and medical students interviewing patients. The students can learn what works and what does not work and how to hone in on a patient's concerns.

Role-modeling has an enormous impact in medical education. We typically mirror our mentors. If they do procedures a certain way, the students naturally follow suit. In past generations, some of our mentors were not very effective communicators, and those skills were passed on to the next generation. However, it is no longer "business as usual," and patients should not tolerate poor communication from their primary caregivers.

It's our job to help our patients talk about what concerns them during an exam-room interaction. Because of embarrassment, patients may be reluctant to talk about their inability to achieve an orgasm or an erection and may visit the doctor under the pretext of having a "cough" or "feeling tired." A good medical "listener" will help the patient get to the important reason why they have come to see a doctor—long before the doctor attempts to leave the room.

We physicians need to be detectives. Patients may not always tell us what we need to know. Therefore, we take clues from the patient's eye contact, body language and voice inflection. And other indicators we can observe and even smell give us clues.

If a patient complains of a cough, for example, and admits to being a heavy smoker, the astute clinician may put two and two together and investigate the cough more thoroughly. A pack of cigarettes in the patient's pocket is another sign, as is a strong smell of cigarette smoke. Suspecting something more serious than a simple cough, the careful doctor may order appropriate tests, such as a CT scan. On the other hand, the busy, hassled doctor with mediocre observation and interviewing skills may miss this opportunity to detect an important condition and send the patient away with a prescription for a cough medication.

What makes patients happy?

Go into your exam with a very clear understanding of your concerns. What is the symptom? You don't have to know all the medical terms. Just tell the doctor exactly what's going on. It is helpful to write down these cues because, under the pressure of time and with the stress of being in a medical environment, patients sometimes forget these sorts of details.

Patients need the support and encouragement of family members and friends. If you bring someone to your exam with you, please make it clear that they should observe but not insert their own prejudices and concerns. After all, they are not the patient. Your needs come first. The patient should sit next to the doctor, and there should not be a family member between the patient and the doctor. This is a symbolic intrusion.

It is also important for the doctor to end the interview with the following statement: "Are there any other concerns? Are there any other issues? Are there any other things that we did not touch on?" This signals you that the medical assessment is coming to a close.

Did you ever try to have a conversation with someone who simply wasn't listening? It's difficult at best. Both verbal and nonverbal cues tip you off to problems in communication or lack of it. During office visits, doctors can either engage you with good listening and communication skills or completely turn you off.

Researchers from the University of North Carolina, writing in the *Journal of the American Board of Family Practice*, looked at ways doctors can improve communication with their patients and whether those techniques improved patient outcomes.

Their findings showed that satisfied patients remembered what the doctor said, were satisfied with the office visit, intended to comply with the treatment and felt trust in the doctor. In the long-term, these patients had improved quality of life. So what did these doctors do to make their patients happy?

The doctors showed empathy and gave reassurance and support. The visits tended to be longer, and the doctors spent more time taking the patient's medical history and explaining treatment options. They used humor and focused on the patient's feelings and emotions. The successful doctors with happy patients also spent time on health education. They shared information in a friendly way and summarized their discussion.

Nonverbally, the better communicators were perceived to show interest in the patient by nodding their heads and leaning forward—all outward signs of attention. They uncrossed their legs and arms and showed they were listening with their body language.

No magic. Simple as that.

The expert listener typically faces the patient, makes solid eye contact, and is not distracted by perhaps children in the examination room or by pagers, beepers or knocks on the door. This is your time, and it should not be diluted by distractions. I personally bristle when I am with a physician (when I am the patient), and the physician answers the pager or picks up the telephone. None of us is getting the Nobel Prize, so to wait fifteen or twenty minutes to answer a phone call certainly will not cause the crumbling of the Western world as we now know it. Expect your doctor to listen, to lean forward with an attentive posture, and occasionally write down comments and concerns.

Another practice that is important is the formal washing of the hands. This signifies that the physical exam is about to begin and is a gesture of respect for the patient—not to mention hygienically appropriate.

In choosing a doctor, you need to feel a positive chemistry. There needs to be the sense that the physician does care for you—the patient—and is concerned about your welfare. Obviously, complete disclosure and honesty and a free sharing of information is crucial. This should be viewed as a partnership, as a relationship to safeguard your health and, if necessary, to rally against a common foe: disease, illness or infirmity.

Male or female doctor—does it matter?

The decision to select a male or female physician is a very personal one. In general, most studies suggest that women are more comfortable with female physicians, and that is certainly understandable. One of my best friends is a very prominent oncologist in an upper Midwestern city, and his primary health-care provider is a woman. He finds that she listens to him, is sensitive to his concerns and thoroughly assesses his condition.

Gender does make a difference though. Female primary-care doctors tend to spend more time with their patients (two minutes more, on average) and engage in more active partnership communication than male physicians, according to a study in *The Journal of the American Medical Association*. Researchers at Johns Hopkins looked at studies comparing male and female doctors for the past thirty years. At the beginning of this chapter, I introduced the one question doctors should always ask but rarely do: How are you feeling? The female doctors, according to research, engage in more emotional discussion around that question, although both male and female doctors delivered similar medical information.

What role does race play? It turns out that you're more likely to be satisfied with your doctor if you and the doctor are the same race, according to research also at Johns Hopkins and published in the *Journal of Health and Social Behavior*. The researchers speculated that patients, when they have a choice, will choose doctors of their same race because they are more likely to trust and feel greater comfort with such doctors. There may be an intrinsic sense of connection. Already you can see we will need many more doctors from various racial and ethnic groups to serve our growing populations.

If it's important to be seen by a doctor of your own race, then by all means factor that into your selection process. A satisfied patient is much more likely to comply with treatment, to keep follow-up appointments and, although doctors won't admit it, less likely to bring a malpractice suit in the event of a problem or bad medical outcome.

This begs the question: What makes a good doctor? What qualities are you looking for in choosing a doctor? Qualities of empathy and sensitive communication are far more important than gender or race.

The bottom line is that patients, no matter their gender or their doctor's gender, want to be listened to. In effect, the patient is saying, "Make me feel important."

My message to you is this

If the chemistry between you and your doctor is not positive, if the energy is not positive, you certainly have the right to request and seek another physician, especially if you have been assigned one by your managed-care provider. This can be done very discreetly, is a common practice and is clearly your right.

Inside the Exam Room

Imagine you're sitting in the exam room, the doctor comes in, says hello, and asks how to help. Imagine you begin speaking and talk until you are finished. The doctor doesn't interrupt. How long do you think most patients will talk if they are not interrupted?

Researchers reporting on a study in the *British Medical Journal* tried just that. Doctors were asked to time their patients using a hidden stopwatch and not interrupt until the patient said something like, "What do you think, doctor?"

The average talk time was just ninety-two seconds, and most patients (78 percent) finished within two minutes. Older patients tended to talk longer. The doctors felt that their patients were providing important information and did not feel the need to interrupt. But that was a forced study.

In actual practice, doctors interrupt in about twenty seconds.

Unless you talk fast, it is absolutely crucial that you have the opportunity to voice your concerns without being shortchanged by the physician jumping in. If the physician interrupts you, I think it is appropriate to say,

"Doctor, I appreciate your jumping in, but please let me finish this thought." This is a reasonable gesture to clearly get your points out on the table.

Should you make and take a list with you? Only a short one, unless you already sent your doctor a note a few days before your appointment. Your doctor will appreciate it if you are organized. There are a few other things you might consider taking with you: a pen and paper and a friend. Please write down what the doctor says. It's perfectly acceptable, and I encourage it. Better yet, your friend can take notes while you engage in a dialogue with the doctor. Of course, this works best if you are comfortable bringing your spouse or sister or caring friend, but many people are not at ease with this.

The down side is that a well-meaning family member or friend can interfere with the doctor–patient relationship by attempting to show off newly found medical knowledge from the Internet or inserting his or her own medical story into the conversation. But the up side is that you will remember (together) what the doctor said—and understand it.

Often, I see patients accompanied by many family members. This may seem unusual, but I'm seeing my patients in a clearly difficult time. They usually have a very serious, life-threatening illness, and their support group is an essential part of their treatment. Everyone has to be on board, and the patient has called upon them to help in the decision making.

Routine exams, however, usually can be handled alone, but feel free to take notes and to ask the doctor to repeat information you didn't hear or don't understand. Some practical and reasonable questions may be these:

- What is my diagnosis? What's going on with me?
- What treatment do you suggest? What are my options?
- What should I be doing now to manage this condition?
- Where can I find out more about my condition?

If you are given a prescription, it's sensible to ask these questions:

- What is this medication and what symptoms does it treat?
- How much do I take, when, and how do I take it?
- What are the possible side effects?
- How will I know if it is working?
- Does this drug interact with any other medications I am taking?
- What should I do if I forget to take it?
- How much does it cost? (If too much, is there an appropriate substitute?)

Your pharmacist can respond to some of these questions about medication, but the best person to ask first is your doctor. Don't wait until you're home from the pharmacy to read the label or printout that comes with your prescription. If you have questions, or you can't remember what the doctor said, call the doctor's office. The doctor's nurse should be able to get answers and get back to you.

The best strategy is not to leave the exam room until you are satisfied that you understand what's going on with you and what you need to do next. A study reported in the *British Medical Journal* concluded that most patients fail to discuss items bothering them and leave with unanswered questions. The result was that the patients were given unnecessary medications, and they didn't stick with their treatment plans.

In this particular study, patients still had questions about symptoms, about prescriptions, and about ways they had tried to self-treat their conditions. They had questions about their diagnoses and wanted to talk about side effects of medications. Such unmet needs may trigger yet another doctor's appointment when you might easily have wrapped up your questions the first time if you had been forthright and fully prepared.

What patients want (and need) to hear

Whatever brings you inside a doctor's exam room, you know what you want to hear from the doctor, and if you don't get answers, reassurance and education from your physician, you will not think you have had a successful medical interaction. Never mind that you may not comply with treatment or that you will call the doctor later if your condition gets worse.

One concerned mother took her son to a dermatologist to find out about some white spots on his face. From start to finish, from the time the doctor walked into the exam room, the entire interaction took less than one minute, and during that time, the doctor said, "Don't worry, Mom," four times.

He glanced at the child, dashed off a prescription, stuck it in her hand and dashed out the door, leaving a frustrated mother with an impatient five-year-old sporting white spots on his face, and a host of unanswered questions.

Sound familiar?

The problem may have been trivial, but the doctor should not have treated it as such. I can guarantee you that the mother may not seek help for another alarming rash that could be more serious. And she certainly won't return to this doctor for treatment ever again.

What the mother needed to hear was this: "Nothing serious, it's just a blah blah blah, and it will go away on its own in two weeks. If not, call me. You can put this cream on it to help it go away faster. We're not sure why these things appear, but it's not contagious."

With this ideal answer, the doctor could have anticipated questions and answered them and still been out the door in maybe two minutes. "Don't worry" was a poor substitution for solid information. And I don't care how much of a hurry the doctor is in, how many calls are on hold and patients backed up sitting in little rooms or if the waiting room is packed with impatient patients reading old magazines, we doctors owe you our time and attention—that's our job. First and foremost, you're the patient. You can decide if you want to worry. The point of honest answers to your questions is to allay your fears.

Some patients go to the doctor with the expectation that they will be given a prescription and everything will be just fine—as if drugs could fix just about anything. Research shows that patients who expected medication were nearly three times more likely to receive a prescription, according to a study in the *British Medical Journal*. When the doctor thought the patient expected medication, the patient was ten times more likely to receive it.

That's why patients are walking out of clinics everywhere with prescriptions for antibiotics when what they have is a viral infection or common cold that a little chicken soup could help (but that's discussed in the next chapter). Antibiotic resistance is a growing concern simply because patients are asking for these potent medications, expecting a prescription, and doctors are complying even when they know a patient won't be helped with it—just because doctors are afraid to send a patient out the door empty-handed. How about filling their minds with information? After all, knowledge is powerful medicine.

Asking for specific medications is a concern because we are seeing an increase in what is called direct-to-consumer drug advertising on TV and in print media. Compelling ads for Viagra or for the "purple pill" are driving you to ask your doctor specifically for them. I've seen prescription fulfillment numbers as high as 30 percent, indicating that doctors are giving patients the medications they are asking for—whether they are appropriate or not. That's the downside.

On the up side (and I do refer here again to Viagra), patients motivated by TV commercials can become more active in their treatment. If a news item or drug commercial opens a dialogue between you and your doctor, all the better. A wise practitioner will seize that teachable moment to discuss your complete health picture and, I hope, take time to explore all your options. Requests for Viagra are getting men into doctors' offices in record numbers. With such newly motivated patients, smart doctors are taking blood pressures and getting cholesterol levels and PSA tests. And dispensing prescriptions for Viagra, if appropriate.

Patients listen when doctors prescribe a healthy lifestyle

Often lost in the doctor–patient dialogue are matters of lifestyle choice. The whole notion of shared decision making is forgotten in that seven-minute encounter. Other patients are waiting. The phones are ringing. Time is ticking away. Who has time to talk about quitting smoking or losing weight?

But it's critical for doctors to take time and make time to counsel you on lifestyle issues—whether you are there for that type of information or not—simply because people trust the doctor's advice more than any other source, and because a doctor's advice changes behavior.

The U.S. Preventive Services Task Force, in a May 2002 report published in the *American Journal of Preventive Medicine,* said, "The unabated impact of health-damaging behaviors among Americans makes it imperative that health-care providers and health-care systems seriously consider these behavioral issues [tobacco use, obesity, lack of exercise] and accept the challenge of routinely providing quality behavioral counseling interventions where proven effective."

I couldn't say it better. The report says that personalized advice from a doctor about breaking bad habits or adopting a healthier lifestyle enhances the patient's motivation to change, which may be that extra behavior-change push from precontemplation (discussed in the earlier chapters) into contemplation and action stages.

Because half of the top-ten causes of death are linked to behaviors such as smoking, inactivity, poor diet, alcohol misuse and obesity, the federal task force has suggested that doctors may even convey health messages phrased like this: "As your physician, I feel I should tell you . . ." as a subtle yet powerful way of engaging you—the patient—in shared decision making.

Can these messages make a difference? Researchers at the University of Wisconsin-Madison wanted to know what happens if doctors talk to their patients a few minutes about drinking habits. Alcohol contributes to liver disease, cancer, problems with developing fetuses in pregnant women, and it's a leading cause of domestic violence, child abuse, accidents and injury. A worthy target for intervention.

Patients aged eighteen to sixty-five who were seeing doctors on routine visits were given a screening questionnaire to look at their at-risk alcohol behaviors. Those who screened positive—meaning they had risky alcohol behaviors such as drinking alone or admitted to drinking too much at times —were given two 15-minute face-to-face conversations with their doctors, followed by two 5-minute phone calls from a nurse. Discussions centered on what was acceptable drinking behavior and how to monitor drinking habits.

Short-term results are always encouraging, but it's the long-term behavior change that truly makes a difference, and it did in this experiment, published in the journal *Alcoholism*. The study participants were followed up over a period of years. Early intervention by the family doctor made a huge difference, even four years after the doctor–patient discussion, by reducing alcohol-related illness and injury.

The bottom line is that it's cost-effective for doctors to spend a few minutes talking with new patients—and with established patients—about their alcohol habits, and up to 20 percent of patients will significantly decrease their alcohol use. In doing so, they lower their risk for accidents and overall health-care costs. It's also important for doctors to discuss alcohol use for another reason: If the doctor is going to prescribe any medication, the doctor needs to know what other medications you are taking and whether you might be in danger of alcohol–drug interactions—and many of these can be serious.

Smokers are tough. Sometimes it seems our nonsmoking messages are falling on deaf ears, but a study at Case Western Reserve University showed that smokers welcome counseling about smoking cessation from their family doctors. In fact, they are more satisfied with their physician visits if the doctors provide this type of counseling. And it's more than just "you need to stop smoking." This study (in *Preventive Medicine*) showed that talking about smoking for as little as three minutes was likely to be effective.

Equally important, in my opinion, is for doctors to give you advice about physical activity. The Surgeon General promotes thirty minutes of activity on most days of the week. Others say sixty minutes is better, but the truth is that 70 percent of our patients are underactive, and that includes their children. This decline in activity is certainly attributed to television and computers, all leading to a steep rise in obesity, type 2 diabetes, colon cancer and high blood pressure. These chronic conditions often don't appear until middle-age, but they have their roots in childhood.

The family physician is perfectly positioned to provide counseling about physical activity, and a study by one of my colleagues at Mayo Clinic, published in the *Mayo Clinic Proceedings,* calls for doctors to literally jump in and "prescribe" exercise. Only half of patients receive advice from their doctors to get moving and to increase their levels of activity. It's time for doctors to write prescriptions for a healthy life in an attempt to tear our patients away from keyboards and TV remotes, get them to walk away from the refrigerator and fast food, and encourage them to be active.

The authors of the study contend that the medical community should lead the way with aggressive counseling simply because the family doctor is almost always the most trusted and authoritative source for health recommendations.

A recent study at several medical centers including the Cooper Clinic (a leader in exercise research) showed just how powerful a little doctorly advice about exercise can be. Participants who received just eighteen minutes of health education boosted their activity levels and lowered their risk for illness. Powerful medicine.

A little doctorly advice goes a long way

Here's another area in which we can do better: Doctors fail to tell women of childbearing age to take a multivitamin containing folic acid to prevent birth defects if they become pregnant, according to a March of Dimes study. Most women still don't know that folic acid must be taken *before* pregnancy to prevent certain defects in newborns. Prevention works. Patients hear and heed lifestyle messages. I hope your physician is riding the white horse of patient education.

Yet the fact of the matter is that doctors do a poor job of providing information (in person and in written educational materials), according to researchers in the Center for Cost and Outcomes Research at the University of Washington-Seattle, writing in the *British Medical Journal.*

Too often, medical decisions fall into a gray area where the best choice for any individual may be unclear and where reasonable people might choose differently. Common examples are certain procedures for back pain or treatment for benign prostate problems. Which drugs to choose for treatment is another gray area, where risks, benefits and side effects need to be weighed.

These types of decisions are made daily in doctor's offices; nevertheless, many questions remain. If you are to become an empowered patient, you must go into the medical arena armed with information (or know where to get the best decision-making tools) because you simply cannot expect to get that from your doctor.

Older patients tend to defer medical decisions to the doctor (this generation still thinks the doctor knows best). But that does not mean these older patients are happy with their treatment. Research in the *British Medical Journal* demonstrated that factors such as knowledge of risk, the doctor's ability to communicate, and the doctor–patient relationship are critical to informed choice. The goal is to get to informed choice yourself and not rely solely on the doctor to get you there, because the doctor simply can't.

Internet changes the doctor–patient relationship

The lifestyle and health decisions you make can mean the difference between life and death—yours. You want the best opinions and the most current and trusted medical advice. If not at your doctor's office, then where can you find it? You *can* get good medical advice on the Internet, but you have to be a savvy shopper and use it to help you, not hurt you.

A gentleman patient of mine from Iowa nearly died because his wife purchased what she thought was a safe "immune-system stimulant" through an unofficial alternative-medicine-type Web site. We were treating him for a brain tumor. She was desperate. Her husband was quite ill. She felt she was helping boost his immune system that was so severely weakened by his condition and his treatment.

Here's what happened: He almost bled to death because of the drug interaction with the bogus substance she found online. Rather embarrassed and certainly concerned, they admitted what they had done. I quickly searched the Internet using a simple search engine and found out what was really in the so-called miracle cure. It was a blood thinner, and in no way was it an immune-system stimulant.

The Internet can work for you and against you. It is a double-edged sword that can have catastrophic complications. The lesson of this story is to work with your doctor and pharmacist to check all drug interactions. Anything you put into your body should be considered in relation to everything else.

Here's another example: One of my patients developed a very rare cancer of the abdominal tissue. An unsophisticated Internet search by the desperate patient uncovered a physician in Miami who was advertising for patients. He was performing surgery on people with this condition. She was practically packed and ready to go when we discussed that surgery was not an option for her situation.

My best advice is to stick with credible medical sites sponsored by major medical institutions such as Johns Hopkins, Harvard, Stanford, Mayo Clinic, and the Web sites operated by health-serving organizations such as the American Cancer Society and the American Heart Association. I refer you to the extensive resource section in the back of this book.

Point, click, heal

Both of the examples above show how the Internet is changing the doctor–patient relationship. Our patients are turning to the Internet to access the very same medical information we have been reading in journals. These patients are coming to the exam room able to begin their medical discussion at a higher level of understanding, and they are changing the way we practice.

Survey after survey still confirms that patients trust information from their doctors more than they trust information from the Internet and other sources such as TV, books and magazines. Rather than undermining our efforts, the Internet can enhance the relationship, but doctors must help patients get to the best, most trusted places on the Internet, or they will spend precious time discussing treatments that are not appropriate for the patient sitting in front of them with a bag full of computer printouts.

The solution, perhaps, is for doctors to direct patients to trusted Internet sites by providing an annotated handout or to set up their own Web sites with links to approved information centers, and certainly there are plenty of well-reviewed and well-written consumer-health information sources on the Internet. The danger lies in a patient conducting a Google search and ending up in uncharted territory. Ask your doctor which Web sites he or she feels comfortable "prescribing." Also consult the resource section at the back of this book.

I recommend you start any Internet search at a portal, megasite or gateway, not at a general search engine such as Yahoo or Google, so you immediately get into a loop of reviewed and trusted sites. Start searches, for example, at a major medical center's megasite such as *MayoClinic.com* or *Intelihealth.com* (a partnership between Harvard Medical School and Aetna). These sites are rich with content on diseases and conditions from A to Z and have decision support tools to help you understand and manage chronic conditions such as migraine or diabetes. You can even sign up for periodic e-newsletters from them.

Other trusted sites to start a search are government portals such as *health.gov, healthfinder.gov* (portals or clearinghouses from which you are directed to content-rich Web sites). I don't discount Web sites funded by educational grants from pharmaceutical companies. Sure, drug companies have a vested interest in the conditions they manufacture drugs for, but they are also robust repositories for information on the condition. They partner with and support nonprofit groups to get the word out. Read their information knowing they have a self-serving interest in your using their medications.

Health-serving organizations are among the best sites to find disease-specific information. The American Heart Association (*americanheart.org*), American Cancer Society (*cancer.org*), American Diabetes Association (*diabetes.org*) and American Lung Association (*lungusa.org*) are nonprofit groups whose sole mission is to gather and convey information on a particular condition. Use them, support them, trust their information.

TEN THINGS TO KNOW ABOUT
EVALUATING MEDICAL RESOURCES ON THE WEB

The federal government's Office on Alternative and Complementary Medicine, among others, has developed guidelines to help you evaluate a Web site.

1. **Who runs this site?**
   Any good health-related Web site should make it easy for you to learn who is responsible for the site and its information. The sponsor should be clearly marked on every major page of the site along with a link to the site's home page. If you can't find the sponsor easily, get outta there.

2. **Who pays for the site?**
   It costs money to run a Web site. The source of a Web site's funding should be clearly stated or readily apparent. For example, Web addresses ending in ".gov" denote a federal government–sponsored site. You should know how the site pays for its existence. Does it sell advertising? Is it sponsored by a drug company? Do you see banner ads or annoying pop-up ads? The source of funding can affect what content is presented, how the content is presented and what the site owners want to accomplish on the site. On the other hand, ads aren't all bad; somebody has to pay for your free access.

3. **What is the purpose of the site?**
   This question is related to who runs and pays for the site. An "About This Site" or "About Us" link appears on many sites. If it's there, use it. The purpose of the site should be clearly stated and should help you evaluate the trustworthiness of the information.

4. **Where does the information come from?**
   Many health/medical sites post information collected from other Web sites or sources. If the person or organization in charge of the site did not create the information, the original source should be clearly labeled.

(continued on following page)

5. **What is the basis of the information?**

   In addition to identifying who wrote the material you are reading, the site should describe the evidence that the material is based on. Medical facts and figures should have references (to articles in reputable medical journals, for example). Also, opinions or advice should be clearly set apart from information that is "evidence-based" (that is, based on research results).

6. **How is the information selected?**

   Is there an editorial board? Do people with excellent professional and scientific qualifications review the material before it is posted? Sites with impressive editorial boards or medical advisory committees eagerly list credentials. Look for these links and look over the group. You want to recognize their academic affiliations.

7. **How current is the information?**

   Web sites should be reviewed and updated on a regular basis (once a year is a good measure). It is particularly important that medical information be current. The most recent update or review date should be clearly posted. Even if the information has not changed, you want to know whether the site owners have reviewed it recently to ensure that it is still valid.

8. **How does the site choose links to other sites?**

   Web sites usually have a policy about how they establish links to other sites. Some medical sites take a conservative approach and don't link to any other sites. Some link to any site that asks, or pays, for a link. Others only link to sites that have met certain criteria.

9. **What information about you does the site collect, and why?**

   Web sites routinely track the paths visitors take through their sites to determine what pages are being used. However, many health Web sites ask you to "subscribe" or "become a member." In some cases, this may be so that they can collect a user-fee or select information for you that is relevant to your concerns. In all cases, this will give the site personal information about you.

(continued on following page)

Any credible health site asking for this kind of information should tell you exactly what they will and will not do with it. Many commercial sites sell "aggregate" (collected) data about their users to other companies—information such as what percentage of their users are women with breast cancer, for example. In some cases, they may collect and reuse information that is "personally identifiable," such as your ZIP code, gender and birth date.

Be certain that you read and understand any privacy policy or similar language on the site, and don't sign up for anything that you are not sure you fully understand. Some health insurers give you a password and access to medical information sites because you are a policyholder. Take advantage of these sites, but use caution about revealing personal health information.

10. **How does the site manage interactions with visitors?**

There should always be a way for you to contact the site owner if you run across problems or have questions or feedback. If the site hosts chat rooms or other online discussion areas, it should tell visitors what the terms of using this service are. Is it moderated? If so, by whom, and why? It is always a good idea to spend time reading the discussion without joining in, so that you feel comfortable with the environment before becoming a participant.

Source: National Center for Complementary and Alternative Medicine (*www.nccam.nih.gov*)

Keep Copies of Your Medical Records at All Times

Unheard of in the past, keeping your own set of records can be truly life-saving. No longer is that manila file in the doctor's office the only place for everything about you, head to toe. Your health records are everywhere. Your family doctor knows when you had your last tetanus shot. The ob/gyn has information on your Pap smear, and the dermatologist has the lab report on the suspicious mole taken off your back three years ago. If you've been in the hospital, inpatient records on your hernia surgery are in their massive record rooms. The walk-in clinic has files on your previous sore throats. And the hospital's emergency department recorded your broken arm or chest pain visit.

Whatever your health status, it's absolutely essential that you gather the pieces of your medical health history and maintain your own master file of medical records.

Why? Because you need them for a number of reasons. First, you need to verify that all information in all your files is accurate, especially regarding information you have told the doctor. I've seen lab reports misfiled, people with similar names getting each other's physician notes, and doctors simply dictating wrong information that is transcribed (or perhaps typed inaccurately) and put into your file.

But why would any of this matter?

- You may need to provide your medical history and past treatment to a new doctor. It would be senseless for a new physician to base treatment decisions on information that was inaccurately recorded or misfiled.
- You might be seeking specialized care from someone like me for a second opinion. We always appreciate knowing the big picture from medical records. I'll give you a life-saving example in a minute.
- Or let's say you are applying for life or health insurance. The prospective insurance company will ask you to sign a release so they can see your medical records. Wouldn't you want to make sure they are correct? You want to monitor what is released and to whom, according to the American Health Information Management Association.

With many different health-care providers, with lab results being faxed and e-mailed, with CT scans digitally transmitted, your personal medical records can be scattered in several doctors' offices, pharmacies and hospitals. And if you have more than one doctor (and most people do), assembling all the essential information in a time of crisis can be a nightmare, if not impossible.

How to gather your records

- **Start your medical record keeping right now.** At your next doctor's appointment, ask for a release form, fill it out, and sign it. Even if there's a small fee, pay it. If you have trouble getting your records, contact your state's department of health. It's your right.

- **Request a copy of everything** including x-rays, reports and correspondence with other doctors. Your doctor is required to make that copy (or might hire a service that will do it for you for a fee) and send records to you.
- **Do this every time you see a doctor** (and specialists) or are in the hospital (pathology reports are helpful if you have surgery) and keep building your records.
- **Track down records** from doctors you've seen in the past and no longer see. Request copies of your records. If doctors have sold their practices, retired or moved to different health-care systems, your records may take some time to locate.
- **Take key records with you** to your appointments in case your file has been "misplaced." If your doctor sees patients in different geographic locations, those paper records are toted around in bins and can easily become lost.

Imagine the horror if you were undergoing treatment for a specific condition or tracking cholesterol, thyroid levels or other blood results from the lab and the doctor's paper file could not be found for comparison. It has happened, believe me.

I had the pleasure of treating a woman whose daughter literally saved her life. When she came to our clinic, she had already seen multiple doctors in many different states. Her daughter kept massive and complete three-ring binders of records during her mother's treatment for a life-threatening illness. When she arrived in my office, I had everything I needed to help her make a life-saving treatment decision, knowing all the efforts and results to date. Otherwise, we would have wasted valuable time and made decisions about treatments that might have already been tried.

During a routine check-up, another patient looked fine except for a spot the size of a nickel on her lung, which was revealed on a chest x-ray. We were naturally suspicious, and everything was moving toward major surgery. Somehow, we were able to find a previous physician who had given her an exam fifteen years ago. The chest x-ray taken then showed the same spot. Then there was no need for surgery, but we wouldn't have known that unless we had the earlier records to compare.

Outcomes for you may not be so critical, but there are times when having an earlier chest x-ray or mammogram (for comparison) or laboratory test results on PSA levels, blood counts, thyroid or liver functions, or adult immunizations can make a critical difference in whether you need treatment or not.

The PSA test (a blood test to screen for prostate cancer) of a sixty-five-year-old patient was 3.7. No problem, right, because normal is in a range between 0 and 4. Most doctors would say, "Thanks for coming, see you next year." But this patient brought along records showing that just a year earlier his PSA was 1, meaning his blood levels had increased fourfold in just one year. So even though he was within a normal range, we arranged a biopsy, caught the cancer early and cured it with surgery. Without his records, he would have been a year farther down the road toward prostate cancer.

Another of my patients showed a very low hemoglobin (a sign of anemia), and we became concerned, until we examined the medical records and took note of his heritage. Hemoglobin is a measure of the red blood cells and their ability to carry oxygen throughout the body. His was 9, and normal is 14 to 16. Fortunately, we had available to us his medical records for the past thirty years. We all breathed a sigh of relief when we saw that he had been at 9 for years. That, coupled with the fact that he was of Italian descent, turned an abnormality into nothing. Mediterranean people can often have DNA blood conditions that would produce these readings.

Until Internet medical record-keeping systems become accessible to any doctor anywhere, with your permission, or until we each wear our medical records on a tiny computer chip inside a bracelet or necklace, we're stuck dealing with paper records scattered in every doctor's office and hospital we've ever been in from birth.

A one-place-for-all-records system in cyberspace is coming. "It's all about empowering the consumer," predicts Tom Ferguson, a physician and online health-industry expert. "There's a clear shift in control to the patient," he says, "with an entirely new concept of patient-owned and patient-controlled records that only you can allow access to."

Until then, take control of your paper records.

Certain key medical records should be with you **at all times.** For example, keep a copy of your EKG—that's a heart tracing—in your wallet or purse if you have any heart problems. Ask your doctor for what we call a rhythm strip. It's a piece of paper about three feet long and three inches high. Simply fold it to about the size of a credit card.

Let's say you show up in the ER with chest pain, and doctors run an

EKG. Let's make this interesting. You're on vacation, hundreds of miles from home. You'll get much better treatment and have a higher chance for faster and accurate treatment if doctors can compare the two readings.

If you're traveling, put this key medical record in your travel bag or brief-case. I also advise my patients who have an abnormal chest x-ray to ask us for a miniature version (about eight by eleven inches). This might show a piece of shrapnel or a bullet that could not be removed. Some metal detec-tors in airports and sensitive venues will pick up these images, and you will need to explain them. You might also wear this information on a medical alert medallion or bracelet.

How you can protect your privacy . . . from doctors who may not even know they're violating it

Your medical information is sensitive, confidential, and just between you and your doctor. But because your medical records are no longer stored just in those familiar manila files in your doctor's office, your personal medical data may instantly be dispatched around the world electronically by fax or e-mail.

Unless you take proper precautions, your private medical information may not be safe. Talk with your doctor and the office staff about ways to preserve your privacy:

- **In person:** Discuss your privacy concerns. People most concerned about preserving privacy may have a family history of a dread disease they want to keep confidential, especially from employers. Most of us would want to keep confidential any issues involving sexually trans-mitted diseases, including HIV/AIDS, pregnancy and mental illness. Find out your doctors' office policies on releasing information and make sure you understand them and agree. If you don't want medical information released for insurance reimbursement, don't sign a release. Pay the entire amount yourself.

- **By voice mail:** The very fact that you are seeing a doctor is confi-dential. The biggest concern is that someone other than you will inter-cept a phone message at home or at work from your doctor's office. Sensitive medical professionals will leave only a basic message, such as "This is Heidi calling for Mrs. Johnson. Please call me at 765-4321." If you have specific wishes about where and how the medical staff may leave a message for you about test results or follow-up, or just to make an appointment, make sure the instructions get recorded on your medical chart.

- **By e-mail:** We are clearly in the age of the virtual or digital office. Without question, e-mail is subtly changing the landscape of medical practice. However, there are some major concerns. First, confidentiality. There is no such thing as a secure browser, and delicate, sensitive and revealing medical information could wind up in the wrong hands. Patients may be denied life insurance or health insurance based upon an intercepted e-mail, and this clearly has to be kept in place. If you e-mail your doctor, don't expect him or her to e-mail you back with information on medical treatment. In order to make an informed diagnosis, your doctor must examine you, and that can't be done by e-mail. Use e-mail only to set up appointments or to obtain referrals.
- **By fax:** If you're expecting a fax of, say, lab results, from your doctor and you use a shared fax machine, set up a time beforehand, by phone, with the doctor's office. Confirm your incoming fax number and baby-sit the fax machine until your fax arrives.
- **By mail:** It's okay for your doctor to notify you by mail (many do) with test results or reminders about upcoming appointments, but you also have the right to request a phone call instead.

Reviewing and amending your records

As a patient, you have an absolute right to review your medical records—and to get a copy. Some medical office staff may resist your request. They simply aren't used to patients asking to see their records. You may ask to see the original file in your doctor's office, but you cannot take it with you. The medical record itself is the property of the doctor.

- Review your file in the doctor's office where medical staff can explain any technical medical terminology and abbreviations. Ask the doctor to correct any information about you that is wrong. Or write a letter to be inserted into your file to clarify any errors or to express your opinion. Make sure the records show your family medical history and emergency numbers, current medications, allergies, organ donor wishes and advance directives.
- Make sure your file is complete and that all information is about *you*— not about somebody with the same or similar name.
- Check and update your health-insurance information, if necessary,

and examine the date of all authorizations you have signed to release medical information—to whom and for what. Change or delete as appropriate.

New federal regulations, outlined by the U.S. Department of Health and Human Services, safeguard the privacy of your medical records. As a patient, you are assured access to your records, and only you can give (or deny) permission for your medical information to be shared with anyone else, including health and life insurers.

How Healthy Is Your Family Tree?

What you don't know about your family tree can cost you your life. On the other hand, knowing your family health history can be empowering and may help you ward off medical problems. No medical record is complete without a family health history.

Does it really matter how Aunt Louise died or whether Grandpa William had a heart condition? Yes.

We know that 10 to 15 percent of people with colon cancer have a family history that includes this disease. If one or both of your parents are alcoholics, we know that 25 percent of their children are at risk for becoming alcohol abusers themselves. Diabetes and high blood pressure also run in families and pose a risk.

You're not doomed to develop diseases just because they are present in your family. And certainly lifestyle, as I have discussed, plays a large part in disease development. With knowledge, you become more vigilant with your lifestyle habits and early health screening.

At your next family reunion, find out about your blood relatives' health histories—how they died, if they were overweight, or had any unusual or unexplained illnesses. It may save your life.

Here's a typical case: A thirty-year-old woman feels just fine but notices a dimpling of one nipple. It looks different from her other breast. In most cases, if she calls it to the attention of her doctor, she'd receive a physical exam and that might be it. Nothing to worry about. But if she mentions that her aunt is undergoing chemotherapy for breast cancer, the stakes are higher. She'd then have a mammogram, maybe an ultrasound and MRI. Her family history of breast cancer raises the index of suspicion. It's not that conscientious doctors would miss the opportunity to find and treat an early condition, but they are busy, and overworked, and the unusual is not always on their radar screen. If you're the patient, say, "Doctor, let me tell you about my family history." That'll get the doctor's attention and get you the proper treatment.

If Aunt Louise died under unusual circumstances and nobody is really sure how she died—and it was years ago—some clues might help you. If the story at the family reunion is that she never woke up from an operation, it could be she was particularly vulnerable to anesthesia. And you might be, too. If you're a blood relative, I'd make sure you told your doctor about this and especially your anesthesiologist if you're scheduled for surgery. In these cases and with certain surgeries, you would be quite closely monitored, and you might elect to have a spinal block instead of general anesthesia. Simple, life-saving.

Map your family health history back to your grandparents, aunts and uncles, great aunts and uncles, first cousins and, of course, your parents and brothers and sisters. Important details, if available, are their gender, year of birth and death, illnesses they may have had and ongoing health conditions, age they were diagnosed, and the cause of their death. Note lifestyle factors such as whether they smoked or were overweight.

You need to gather and safeguard your medical records and those of your children. Keep your family health history with your medical records. Know as much about your family medical history as you can. Someday, those records may make the difference in life-saving medical decisions.

My Thoughts . . .

I advise you to go into the exam room fully prepared to make your all-too-brief encounter highly productive. Don't let anything deter you from your mission—not the doctor's pager, a friend's off-track questions, weird stuff from the Internet, or trivial concerns that take time away from the big issues that brought you to the doctor in the first place. What is your mission? You are seeing a health-care professional for a very specific medical question, whether this is a pain, a worry or a routine exam.

Your doctor should give you the courtesy of letting you explain your concerns in your own terms. Don't let the doctor jump in until you have had a chance to tell your story—and typically this takes only a few minutes. In other words, you are there to tell your story and to be listened to.

As clinicians, we can look at records and x-rays and test results, but we need to hear the rest of the story—and that can only be done by carefully listening to our patient.

Your obligation as a patient is to come prepared for an exchange of information. Your preparation must include knowing your medical history, and that means having medical records available. Unheard of in the past, it's not unusual at all for someone to assemble their own complete medical record.

Most parents keep track of their children's immunizations faithfully because schools and camps need this information. So it's a natural extension to track a thyroid level or cholesterol or blood pressure. You want to know these numbers as they increase or decrease over a period of time. From one doctor visit to another, you may move cities or see different doctors. Doctors don't have a central clearinghouse for information about every person (at least not yet, although the Internet poses some promising innovations). Until then, the only person who can maintain continuity of care for you is *you*.

Medical records are your property—at least the information contained in them. They are part of you. You are entitled to copies of everything about you. You are also entitled to an explanation of your records, and it is appropriate for you to ask your care provider for clarification.

Armed with your own medical history and a sense of empowerment to make the medical-care system truly care for you, you can enter any exam room prepared to talk so your doctor will listen.

9

What They Never Taught Me in Medical School

Time is generally the best doctor.

—Ovid

Mark McCormick is a genius. He is a sports entrepreneur who recognized in the 1960s the interest that we Americans have for celebrities. McCormick knew that golf would play a major role in American leisure sports, and the gentleman of great affection at that time was Arnold Palmer. So McCormick developed a relationship with Mr. Palmer and acted on his behalf. A spinoff from those days was a book entitled *What They Don't Teach You at Harvard Business School.* The book had some excellent advice from a street-smart and savvy negotiator rather than the typical material you'd find in a business-school handbook.

This type of insider advice is invaluable—in medicine. Much of what we do as physicians has very little to do with what we were taught in medical school. The street-smart stuff, well, we learn that later—sometimes the hard way. Let me give you some examples of what we were *not* taught in medical school—but stuff I know after years of practicing medicine:

- **Patients want to be acknowledged and listened to.** That means it is not good form for your doctor to respond to interruptions, such as a phone call, knock on the door or pager. Doctors should put these distractions off for several minutes. It causes no harm. If your doctor is interrupted, make it clear that you do not want to be left in the lurch again. Emergencies are understandable of course, but rare.

- **Most patients have difficulty following treatment instructions.** Especially if you're talking with your doctor about an emotionally charged diagnosis, such as cancer or another life-changing condition, you may not remember what you discussed. Even for small office procedures, such as removal of a mole, patients don't remember their wound-care instructions—thus jeopardizing healing. I advise you to take notes, ask the doctor to repeat something if you didn't hear it, ask for clarification if you don't understand it, and follow up with phone calls to the doctor if you have any confusion, especially about medication. You are perfectly welcome to invite pertinent family members or close friends to sit in on the discussions. I foresee the day when physicians will prescribe information. Yes, information. Instead of handing our patients a brochure, which without verbal instruction is not good form, Web-savvy doctors will follow up by sending patients an e-mail with informative links back to the doctor's Web site. If your doctor doesn't have a Web site with information, ask if the doctor recommends any particular sites where you can read more about your condition or procedure.

- **If you can see it, you can understand it.** Most patients and families are fascinated by x-rays, CT scans and bone scans. You are entitled to see what your imaging studies look like. By seeing the broken wrist or breast tumor, you can visualize what's going on with you. These pictures really are worth a thousand words when it comes to understanding your illness or conditions. Ask the doctor to show you your imaging studies and to explain them. Doctors should point out the fractured wrist, the shadow on the mammogram, the blocked coronary artery, the ultrasound shadows.

- **The doctor does not always know best.** Many patients are too frightened to ask questions, and some still believe that the doctor knows best. We don't. But we try to develop a relationship with our patients so that there is a partnership in protecting your health and attacking a common foe if need be.

- **Doctors can make mistakes.** You can guard against being an innocent victim. One woman's x-ray showed a dark shadow on her lung. There was discussion among my colleagues about additional diagnostic testing perhaps leading to major surgery. It wasn't until another doctor carefully examined the patient, including a physical inspection of her chest, and discovered that a thick mole on her breast was the cause of the shadow on the x-ray. The physical exam is so crucial in interpreting any imaging tool, such as x-rays or CT scans. I've seen people tentatively diagnosed with cancer when it turned out the "spots" on the x-rays were the sticky rectangles of a TENS unit (a small box designed to deliver electrical impulses to people with chronic pain). Make sure the doctor looks at *you,* not just at your x-ray.
- **Doctors know how long you'll be in the hospital, even if they tell you they don't.** Patients always ask me, "How long will I be in the hospital?" Doctors try to avoid this one, but they do know. When you are admitted for a diagnosis, there is always a ballpark figure for the number of days for that diagnosis. I think it's important for you to know how long you might be confined because you have to make arrangements for child-care, elder-care, work or feeding the dog. If you can see the end of the tunnel, you can be better prepared. Pin the doctor down and ask, "For someone with my admitting diagnosis, what is the average length of stay in the hospital?" There's always an answer to that question.

Understanding Tradition and Culture

Patients are not simply a medical chart or "the lady in room 2307 with colon cancer." All patients bring to the bedside their culture, their heritage, their history and, perhaps, centuries of abuse, neglect and the results of poverty, war and displacement. Physicians need to understand these issues when treating any patient for any condition. It is especially essential for us to be sensitive to everything about a patient, particularly when we're talking about a life-changing disease.

Mrs. C., for example, was a seventy-three-year-old grandmother from an Asian country who was visiting her family in upstate New York. While in that city, she developed severe back pain. A biopsy revealed an aggressive cancer, which arose from the lung. She had received an appropriate program of radiation therapy at a major medical center and was relatively pain-free. However, because of increasing pain and because of a previous evaluation at the Mayo Clinic, she and her family arrived in Rochester, and I met her in the exam room.

A very careful physical examination demonstrated weakness of the lower limbs, and an MRI scan of the spine demonstrated an obvious tumor pressing on the spinal cord. It was not possible to provide additional radiation therapy without major damage to the spinal cord. Conferences with gifted and compassionate surgeons led to a grim conclusion: Surgery would not be possible because of the extent of the cancer.

We treated her aggressively with steroid medication to decrease swelling around the tumor in the hopes of buying time. Chemotherapy was not appropriate because the tumor was resistant to all known forms of therapy.

That's the medical part.

Mrs. C. spoke no English. The daughter who accompanied her likewise spoke only an Asian dialect. Fortunately, one of our chief residents was fluent in the patient's language, so let me share with you what unfolded.

We learned that it was not appropriate to mention the word *cancer* because the family was fearful that she would "give up and lose all hope." So we acquiesced to the family's wishes and used the word *tumor,* which was quite acceptable. Indeed, we do learn from patients.

When dealing with people from all parts of the world—of which we have very little knowledge—it is always appropriate to ask the responsible family member how some of these issues should be handled. The word *cancer* can have devastating implications in some cultures and needs to be appropriately reframed within the context of sharing with the family the potential seriousness of the situation. This is not deceit; this is appropriate compassion, recognizing the cultural nuances of many patients.

He is the best physician who is the most ingenious inspirer of hope.

—Samuel Taylor Coleridge

The art and science of treatment

We in Rochester have seen a remarkable increase in individuals from the East African region, especially Somalia. These patients bring to the heartland of Minnesota cultures and traditions and histories that are very different from those of the typical Midwesterner. It is not appropriate in some circumstances for a male physician to extend his hand, and it is also not appropriate for discussions to be directed at the female patient. Decisions of a great magnitude typically are filtered through and made by the responsible man of the family who might be a brother, a father or a husband. We need to understand that patients are not always like us. We need to be sensitive to cultural issues and to hone in on how these difficult issues should be addressed in different cultures.

As an institution, we've had great experience with members of the Southeast Asian community. Again, issues of health and wellness are treated very differently among patients from some of those countries. The physician is viewed as the healer with all knowledge of illness. Therefore, it is bizarre to them when physicians inquire and probe to obtain a medical history from the patient. Their expectation is, "I come to you for help. You have all the answers. So why are you questioning me?"

I received a vivid lesson in this during a recent trip to Ireland. I had the opportunity of speaking in the west coast city of Galway. I was impressed how the Irish dealt with the diagnosis of advanced cancer. In most circumstances, the elderly patients had a peace and an acceptance, had belief in an afterlife, and quietly accepted the recommendations of their physicians to treat symptoms and to focus on quality-of-life.

Many patients graciously accepted this news and were prepared to leave the hospital and return home after thanking the caregivers for their guidance and compassion. What a contrast to many American situations, in which I see a frantic race to the airport to fly off and seek the elusive medical Holy Grail when, in fact, time might be more profitably spent at home.

The patient we see today may well reflect hundreds or thousands of years of history, culture and tradition. We need to recognize that some members of our community may distrust traditional medicine. We need to understand this, and we need to walk with the individual and support the decisions with which they are comfortable. No, doctors don't always know best. We learn from our patients every day.

Hospitals Can Be Dangerous
Places—Protect Yourself at All Times

Americans were shocked by the headline: *Being a patient in the hospital can be hazardous to your health*. A national study from the Institute of Medicine reported that approximately ninety-eight thousand patients die each year as a result of medical mistakes made in hospitals. This is one of the first national studies addressing in depth what can happen in a hospital. The report did not address the same kinds of errors that can be committed in other settings, such as your doctor's office and outpatient surgery centers. And the report outlined deaths, not injuries, which are probably even higher.

Obviously, this kind of report generates much concern. The types of errors noted were misread lab reports, blood mismatched during transfusions, wrong prescriptions given to the wrong person or in the wrong dose, and wrong-site surgery, which is removing the left leg or left kidney, for example, when it was the right leg or right kidney (or similarly paired body organ) that was diseased.

Infections acquired in hospitals can be deadly. The CDC says half the infections can be prevented by proper hand-washing. Whose job is it to police the care provider in hand-washing? The patient's? But doctors and nurses wear gloves, you say. Yes, gloves have become ever-present, yet gloves are designed to protect the wearer, not you. Gloves can surely spread germs if they become contaminated, just like a bare hand. Think about it.

What has caused the problem of medical error? There are as many answers as there are experts in this area, but let me take a stab at it. Keep in mind I'm trying to explain some reasons behind this problem, knowing that there is no excuse for medical error.

Medical care is becoming increasingly complex

The body of medical information in scientific research journals is doubling approximately every twenty-four to thirty-six months. New drugs are launched into the marketplace daily. Therefore, it is impossible for any one medical professional to keep up to date with the latest developments. This is especially important when patients receive many kinds of medications, particularly because some of these may interact with each other in dangerous ways.

Patients need to be proactive and clearly understand the dosages, frequencies and the reasons for the medications that they are taking. But patients and families cannot be expected to understand the complex interactions among a variety of medications. This is why physicians, pharmacists and nurses work closely to monitor any bad side effects or interactions, which may occur when medications react to each other inside the body.

Likewise, a clear doctor–patient dialogue should occur about what medications are being prescribed and taken. Rather than add another medication to an already long list, we physicians need to be challenged to reduce medications to the absolute minimum.

You can minimize your risks if you understand what medications you are taking and question any new drugs given to you—especially if you're in the hospital. For example, a single aspirin tablet is well known to interfere with blood clotting for several days, and medications such as the nonsteroidal anti-inflammatory medications (Motrin and Advil, for example) can likewise interfere with blood clotting.

Know what medications you're taking and what they're for. I'm talking about everything in your kitchen cupboard that's loaded with prescription drugs and all kinds of cold and cough remedies you purchased at Wal-Mart. Be aware of their general side effects and also understand the lowest effective dose you can take. New standardized labels on over-the-counter medications are easier to understand, though you'll still have to put your glasses on to read them.

Medical technology makes advances

At the same time medical care is advancing, medical devices are increasing in their complexity. Biopsies are now being performed on parts of the body that were never accessible in the past. Through the techniques of ultrasound-guided biopsies and CT-scan-guided biopsies, tiny pieces of tissue can be extracted from organs such as the pancreas and also from lymph nodes buried deep in the abdominal or pelvic cavities. In the past, some patients required a major abdominal operation to secure this type of tissue.

These procedures can now be performed much more safely. Various types of tubes can be placed into intestinal cavities, and these may pose risks for infection. Intravenous dye tests are now routinely used, whereas formerly, these had been part of medical diagnoses only infrequently. But every invasive test, from the taking of blood to a major operation, poses risks for the patient. Know and understand your risks.

We are becoming a nation of older people

The older person typically does not have just one medical condition but may have many medical conditions, which can be complicated to manage and thus put an older person at higher risk for error. Some older patients are not in as good physical shape as younger patients, and this could complicate any postoperative care. In fact, some patients may be denied chemotherapy, radiation or surgery simply because they are too weak from a chronic medical condition, and the risks of these interventions are too high.

The older person who maintains an excellent level of fitness under most circumstances does not have an increased risk of postoperative complications such as pneumonia, stroke or heart attack. What this means is that the more fit we are and the better care we take of ourselves, the better the odds are that we will be able to withstand the rigors of treatment or the rigors of surgery and obtain the best possible outcome.

We are in the midst of a national shortage of nurses

Some nurses are working back-to-back shifts, and a twelve-hour shift is not at all uncommon. We need to acknowledge that a fatigue factor exists.

Obviously, the patient and the family cannot be expected to make an impact on the national shortage of nurses. However, patients and families can be vigilant and participate with the nursing staff in major decisions. You may (and should) ask the nurse taking care of you why a medication is being given. It is your right to know why a certain test is sensible. If the answers to these questions simply don't feel right or if you have a level of discomfort, it would be prudent to ask for reassurance or clarification from another member of the nursing team.

Another option: If you (or a family member) feel a problem has emerged that will require evaluation in the hospital or in the emergency room, it makes good sense to try to make the visit as early as possible in the day. Realistically, this may not always be feasible because illnesses and accidents don't follow the clock. But if you have the option, it is probably far better to seek medical guidance during the light of day than to walk into the emergency room at three in the morning.

Be an Empowered Patient

Now what can we do about medical error? Some experts are suggesting that we in medicine can learn much from our colleagues in the airline industry. Although the crash of a passenger plane is a catastrophe and makes headlines and the evening news, these events are extraordinarily infrequent. Statistically, flying in an airplane is one of the safest modes of travel. The airline industry has put into place elaborate, consistent and user-friendly protocols, programs and safeguards of checks and double-checks to minimize the human element of error.

The Institute of Medicine has clearly documented that thousands of patients die each year from preventable and avoidable medical mistakes. Programs are now being crafted to monitor this situation, but what can *you* do in the meantime?

- Ask questions. Never assume that everyone taking part in your care knows all the details about you and your medical history, including any allergies or bad reactions—especially to medications.
- Ask about the dosages of each medication and the anticipated duration of treatment when they are prescribed.
- Understand your treatment. For example, some types of chemotherapy are administered over six to eight hours on an outpatient basis. If one of your treatments is completed in two hours rather than six hours, you need to inquire as to why this change in the schedule has occurred.
- If you're in the hospital and a health-care practitioner hands you a pill, don't take it until that person checks your ID bracelet. Imagine what would happen if the person in the bed next to you has the same or similar name. Ask questions: What is this pill? What is this for? If your regular blood pressure pills are yellow and the nurse brings you a blue pill, ask before you swallow. If the technician is hanging a new IV bag with medication or blood, is your name on that bag? Check first.
- Having surgery? Surgeons now are signing their name on the site of your anticipated incision before you are put under anesthesia. If the biopsy is on your left breast, for example, you might even have the nurse write "NO" on surgical tape and place it across your right breast.
- If the doctor writes you a prescription and you can't read it, don't presume that the pharmacist can. Ask the name of the medication, what it is for, and how often you will take it. Confirm all these details with

the pharmacist when you have the prescription filled. And make sure the prescription you are given is for you. Is your name on the bottle? If this is a refill, do the pills look the same as last time?

- From a practical standpoint, understanding what you can expect when entering the hospital as a patient is important. Then you may know if something isn't quite right. Ask questions like: "Do I have to be fasting for certain tests? What will happen to me before surgery and after surgery? Do you expect that I will be receiving blood or antibiotics following surgery or while in the hospital? If so, how much blood will I be receiving? Over what time will it be given? What is the name of the antibiotic, and what is the dose and frequency?"

Patients Have Rights, Too

Your doctor may be in charge of your care when you're in the hospital, but you're still in charge of you. If you're in the hospital as a patient, you *do* have control over what happens to you, even though you may think you're at the mercy of anyone who pokes and prods you. Patients hate to be awakened at four in the morning for a blood pressure reading. They really don't like to be stuck for blood five times a day. Most patients put up with this because they think they don't have control over it.

Well, you do have control. You do have rights. Every hospital has a patient's bill of rights. If you aren't given a copy when you come in, ask for one. Negotiate with the nursing staff and tell them you do not want to be awakened if you are asleep—at any time of day. The lead nurse is your best advocate. Find out who this person is and make sure you both agree that if blood has to be drawn for different doctors, the lab draws it all at once. Bring a family member or friend to be your advocate because you're not on top of your game. Hey, you're in the hospital.

Hospitals have visiting hours, but that's to prevent anyone and everyone from traipsing into your room—and invading your privacy—at any hour of the day or night. Nothing prevents you from having a close friend or family member sitting by your bedside monitoring your activities anytime, helping you with the little things like getting water or changing the TV channel, as long as this person doesn't get in the way of your care. Especially if you're just coming out of anesthesia or are quite weak and unable to truly communicate your needs, I recommend that you have your advocate at your side.

If it were an ideal world, a confidential mechanism of documenting mistakes would exist with constructive and positive steps to avoid them in the future. After all, any one of us on any day may be in a hospital.

In short, be informed and actively participate in your treatment process.

It's sensible to be appropriately inquisitive and proactive and participate with the health-care providers. Ask your targeted questions, such as the ones listed here and elsewhere in this book. During times of high stress and anxiety, it's impossible for any of us to remember what we wanted to ask and then to remember the doctor's answer. That's why I always recommend that an advocate or a family member or a confidante accompany the patient and act on that patient's behalf with the patient's permission.

You will be asked to sign an informed consent sheet for many procedures. You will receive a copy of this form to remind you of the discussions and what you can anticipate about the treatment duration, the possible side effects, and whom to contact if a complication occurs. Don't sign until all your questions are answered.

Patients always have questions about their upcoming procedures or surgery. They want to know when their stitches will be taken out or when they can return to work. We are asked all kinds of questions, and a doctor or other health-care practitioner should be prepared to answer any and all questions patiently. An effortless way out for some health-care providers is to give you easy-to-understand handouts and pamphlets addressing the specifics of many procedures—from appendectomy to vasectomy. Many medical offices have these types of patient-education tools available, even videos.

But for a doctor or other health-care provider to simply hand you a brochure and not be available to answer your questions is not ideal. The informed patient is better positioned to get the maximum benefit from care. The Internet is, of course, changing the information stage, and more information than you ever thought possible is at your command by keystroke. As I've mentioned already, trust only sites maintained by credible organizations and use the information you find to guide your discussions with your health-care providers, not replace them.

Sometimes your morning newspaper or evening TV news may be your source for medical information, and therein may lie a problem.

Don't (Always) Believe the Headlines—Separating Hype from Hope

The cure for cancer is on *The Today Show*. At least that's what you thought you heard. Advances in medical treatment make headline news every day. Local TV anchors do what are called "cut-ins" to tease you to stay tuned for your local news. They'll mention the "new cure for [insert disease name here]" or the "breakthrough treatment that's saving lives." You stay tuned, you listen, and you eventually (maybe) hear that the so-called breakthrough took place in a laboratory rat, and the technology is still years from being tried on humans, if it ever gets that far.

The gap between what's going on in the laboratory and actual clinical practice is huge. Additionally, the media often are quick to latch onto what they think are scientific truths, when, in fact, the science behind "a cure" is evolving slowly and taking its academic time. No one told us in medical school that our patients would challenge us about something they heard on the evening news.

Medical news can be confusing. By the time a clinical study gets into your local newspaper, the information has gone through so many filters, you can't be sure you're getting the whole story. The bottom line for you is the answer to this question: *What does this information mean to me?*

Journalists are wise to avoid charged words such as *breakthrough* and *medical miracle*—although such overblown descriptions are enticing and boost ratings and readership. Words like that should rarely be used in mainstream medical news coverage. Medicine is advancing, but in slow, steady increments. The *cure* for cancer or diabetes or multiple sclerosis is not going to pop into tomorrow's headlines. The forerunner to any cure is happening today in laboratories and in clinics through clinical trials. Preliminary results are written and then circulated to experts in the field. If judged credible, the studies are reported in peer-reviewed medical journals. This process takes months and years, and none of us involved in deliberate medical research would ever characterize our work as a medical miracle. We have many failures you never read about in the headlines.

The only place to read headlines about a cure for cancer or the common cold is in a supermarket tabloid. And while some Internet chat rooms may be abuzz with talk of wiping out the West Nile Virus or Ebola, it's just not going to happen quickly.

The problem comes when journalists misinterpret preliminary findings and make the leap from the laboratory to mainstream medical practice, raising false hopes. Medical breakthroughs are not leaps at all, but slow deliberate steps.

CAN YOU BELIEVE
WHAT YOU READ IN THE HEADLINES?

I suggest you follow these guidelines in evaluating the headlines in the news media and then judge for yourself:

Was the study performed by responsible, credentialed investigators at a major center?

Now don't misunderstand me. Sometimes the obscure researcher in a relatively unheard-of institution may find a key piece of the puzzle. However, that is unusual. So if you do not recognize the name of the institution, university or medical center, or if you do not recognize the credentials of the researcher, you need to be cautious.

Was the vaccine or drug analyzed in a randomized clinical trial?

In other words, were some patients given a vaccine and others given a placebo to sort out whether or not the vaccine really works? Without a test group and a group that receives no treatment or drug, it's hard to say something "works."

How many patients received the treatment?

In order to determine the benefit from a treatment (such as surgery or a drug), it is highly likely that hundreds of patients are needed in a clinical trial. If the number is limited to a dozen or so people with the same disease or condition, you need to be very leery of the results. Were humans used at all, or was this a research study conducted with laboratory rats?

(continued on following page)

Who is the sponsor?

If the press release or the news commentary is exclusively sponsored by a drug company, you need to carefully interpret the data. Our colleagues in the pharmaceutical industry are in partnership with medical practitioners. Few institutions such as medical centers or universities have the resources to conduct research without financial support. We need to cooperate and collaborate with input from the pharmaceutical industry. However, we also need to recognize that we live in the real world and sometimes economic motives may artificially inflate the benefit from the vaccine.

How is the trial conducted?

In other words, every patient who receives the treatment needs to be accounted for. Let's suppose the press release indicated that the benefit occurred in 50 percent of patients who took a flu vaccine. Then the research indicated that five of ten patients received benefit, ten being the total number in the trial. Yet in reality perhaps fifty patients were entered into the trial, so the benefit is really five divided by fifty which equals 10 percent rather than 50 percent. We need to ask the question: What happened to the other forty patients? In other words, there's a difference between the fifty people who entered the study and the ten who were finally analyzed. If every patient is not accounted for, then the interpretation must be suspect.

The pace of medical research can be maddeningly slow, and it is not likely that a researcher laboring in some underground bunker will come forward with the home-run therapy for diseases x, y or z. Science simply does not work like that.

From a cancer perspective let's focus on the interferon story. Approximately twenty years ago, this medication appeared on the cover of *Time* magazine and was heralded as the answer for cancer as well as a whole host of other disorders, such as multiple sclerosis and hepatitis. Study after study carefully addressed the value of this agent, and at the present time, the high hopes for this medication have been disappointing. We now know that interferon can be a toxic medication, and its value applies only to a very small number of patients with some highly unusual diseases. The lesson: We need to be cautious, we need to be somewhat cynical, and we need to be suspicious when a home-run therapy is touted in the news.

Shift gears for a moment and look at coronary artery disease, the number-one killer in America. For decades, medical dogma has clearly focused on the role of cholesterol as a major factor in blocking the arteries. There is rock-solid science that cholesterol is a major factor in causing heart attacks. But hold on, new blood studies are focusing on inflammation as a factor in heart disease and a substance in the blood—C-reactive protein—which may point toward individuals at high risk for a heart attack even if they have a normal cholesterol level. Science is always questioning itself; that's the nature of inquiry.

Consider ulcers. For centuries we believed that ulcers were related to stress and undoubtedly were related to a weakening in the wall of the stomach that allowed acid to erode a hole in the stomach. "Don't get stressed or you'll get an ulcer" was the reasoning. We now know that ulcers are caused by infectious germs—not stress—and antibiotics are part of mainstream therapy for ulcer disease. Stress? I'm not sure where we go with that now. Stress can be hazardous to your health, as we have discussed earlier. For ulcers, however, you'll probably have to blame them on something other than your boss.

So how can we separate hype from actual hope?

Let me take you behind some of the real headlines from mainstream newspapers and magazines (not supermarket tabloids), so next time you read or hear about a so-called cure or other breakthrough, you can judge for yourself.

My favorite story is about nearsightedness. Perhaps you remember it. It was a scary headline: **Nighttime room lighting during infancy linked to nearsightedness.** Oh, the guilt! How could a harmless little nightlight in a child's room lead to babies needing glasses? Well, that's what researchers "suggested" in a study published in a major scientific journal. Or did they?

The researchers had sewn shut the eyelids on monkeys and chickens in laboratories where they slept with bright lights on. Sure enough, the test animals developed eye problems. No real children were harmed in this study!

Of course, no one had checked to see if the monkey and chicken parents needed glasses for vision correction because, frankly, among humans that would be the first thing to be questioned. If your parents need glasses, chances are you will, too. But when the research experiment was reported in sound bites on the evening news, all of a sudden it's not about chickens but about our children, suggesting that bright lighting in their bedrooms may cause the same harmful effect on eyesight.

Imagine the millions of parents ripping out nightlights in their children's rooms.

It's important to evaluate what you read and hear. Consider the source. And even when it comes from a trusted source, you should have clues that the information may be called "preliminary," "suggestive" or "requires further study." Also understand that even established authorities often disagree among themselves about research findings.

Let me give you another chicken story; this one is about chicken soup and the common cold. There's something about chicken soup that just makes you feel better when you're sneezing and sniffling through a winter cold. Is it the loving care Mom provides along with the soup? Could it be the steamy aroma and nutrient-rich broth? Could it be something else?

Scientists at the University of Nebraska Medical Center studied "Grandma's soup"—prepared by the lead researcher's wife from a family recipe—in the laboratory under carefully controlled conditions.

Although common colds are not completely understood, it is believed the inflammation caused when the body defends itself against infection could be blocked by the chicken soup. And that is indeed what Stephen Rennard, M.D., and his colleagues found—*in test tubes.*

If soup can reduce inflammation, which researchers measured in the lab, it *might* reduce the symptoms of a cold. Theory. Speculation. Something to study further.

Results were published by the American College of Chest Physicians in the journal *Chest* and supports what some may see as a food-as-medicine theory. And the headlines proclaimed, of course, that chicken soup cures the common cold. That's not what the scientists found; that's what overly enthusiastic news reporters mistakenly interpreted and put out on the wires. Much of the resultant media frenzy didn't even mention that the findings were restricted to cold germs in test tubes.

The university press relations people had great fun in an out-of-control situation, and as part of their damage control, they put Grandma's soup recipe on the university's Web site. In this case, no damage was done, and people with colds that winter were probably making plenty of chicken soup. Every cold and flu season since, this research gets dragged out and paraded as a "cure." Even if it hasn't been proven to cure anything yet, soup rehydrates the body (warms the soul) and is just plain good for you, especially when you're feeling ill.

Want more?

- Headlines from the University of California-San Diego reported on research published in Proceedings of the National Academy of Science: **UCSD team demonstrates potential for widely effective cancer vaccine.** Patients began lining up for the vaccine. The truth is that there is potential here. But randomized trials are the gold standard, and there are no trials being conducted in this area yet. This study reported on tests done in test tubes in a lab. Sometimes the media make news when it is not ready for prime time.

- Canadian research results presented at the Nutrition, Food and Health Research Centre in London were described in the press: **Pass the tomato juice: It has a substance that may be cancer's master switch.** Wow, let's buy stock in V8. The reality is that cancer is more than two hundred different diseases. Get real. No one switch works for all. And this switch is not proven.

- A University of Portland researcher presented results from a study at the American Chemical Society. The talk was reported in this way: **Researchers find cancer-fighting chemical in hazelnuts.** So that's the secret. We thought the answer was a substance called laetrile found in apricot pits. A Mayo Clinic study proved laetrile's so-called benefits to be negative. Be wary of preliminary study results given in a talk to a professional group. The research has not been peer-reviewed or subjected to scientific scrutiny.

- **Scientists extend life span.** There it is, on the Internet on one of the most highly viewed health Web sites. Here's the first paragraph: "Scientists report finding the fountain of youth—for roundworms. Still, it offers hope for humans." Give me a break. A team of scientists at the University of California tinkered with the genes of roundworms. Turns out humans don't even have the same genes these worms do. This is not news.

- **Low-cal diet keeps heart young.** Grab your attention? Sure, but this is only relevant if you're a mouse. The study at the University of Wisconsin, published in a scientific journal, showed that low-calorie diets helped mice live longer and healthier. How the scientists could make the leap and speculate that "if people reduce their current calorie intake between 20 and 40 percent, even starting in middle age, they may delay the development of heart disease or possibly even prevent it" seems rather bold to me.

Now you and I can look around and see that regulars at the all-you-can-eat buffet are not living into old age. We also know that people who live on the island of Okinawa consume fewer calories than others of us and they tend to live rather long lives. But it would be irresponsible for a scientist to make a definitive statement about humans based on observations on mice. The next step for this research is to test the theories on humans. Done right, this type of research—if proven—could make the headlines years from now.

- But let's pursue the diet question a step further. The low-carbohydrate diet has been as controversial as the butter or margarine question. Do people really lose weight on this diet plan? Of course they do, because the diet calls for you to cut out certain foods and their nutrients, and because all diets work at least in the short-term. Once again we see headlines that the diet works (**Low-carbohydrate diet associated with greater weight loss**), and by the time this book is published, you may see a few more iterations on this theme.

  The most recent presentation was to the scientific session of the American Heart Association in support of the diet's ability to promote weight loss. Let me point out the shortcomings that were not commonly seen behind the headlines: This was a presentation, not a peer-reviewed journal. Therefore, it was not scrutinized by colleagues beforehand. The study involved 120 volunteers—a problem right from the start. Volunteers would not necessarily represent a typical dieter. And when you look at the numbers, most were white women. At 120 subjects, the sample size was small, and there are no long-term data. I'll bet these volunteers have not held their weight loss. So before you start scrambling those eggs and frying the bacon or eating your burgers without a bun, please use good sense and eat sensibly, not according to any restrictive diet.

- The *Los Angeles Times* reported: **Drug aims to inhibit cancer by altering cell environment.** This drug is called Velcade (bortzomid), and its potential use is for patients with multiple myeloma, a type of bone marrow cancer. The initial studies appeared promising, but this usually is the case because patients participating in early clinical trials like this one usually are carefully selected. This particular medication is of great interest because it blocks a series of enzymes that are involved with cell division. In early laboratory studies, this medication induced cell death. However, we must await a long-term study involving hundreds of patients before the verdict is finally in. This item is of interest to me and my medical colleagues but doesn't merit headline news—not yet.

- A press release, dateline New York: **New hope for vaccine to fight rheumatoid arthritis, other autoimmune diseases.** A new vaccine reversed an arthritic-like disease. But the disease was found in rats, not humans. It wasn't until the last paragraph of a two-page press release that researchers said the "next step" was to move toward clinical tests of the vaccine in humans. A small step, no breakthrough.

- Headline news in *The Washington Post:* **Immune cells used to stop severe cancer.** For decades, scientists have been intrigued by the notion of ramping up the immune system to kill cancer cells. While theoretically appealing and scientifically plausible, most of these studies have been disappointing. We must view the initially promising results with appropriate skepticism, fully recognizing that some day we might be able to harness the immune system. But the results to date don't live up to the headline.

- Data from the National Cancer Institute were presented with this headline: **Shark cancers cast more doubt on cartilage pills.** Sharks are supposed to have super immune systems and apparently do not get cancer, so whatever sharks have should be used to treat cancers in humans. Or so the theory went. In this study, government scientists were attempting to disprove the value of shark cartilage as a cancer cure. This study confirms clinical studies at Mayo Clinic and other organizations that show no value from shark cartilage other than to fuel the false hopes of desperate patients. Our results were negative. Shark cartilage has no effect, and apparently sharks do get cancer. Even with major medical centers disproving its value, shark cartilage is still big business. You can do a global Internet search and find hundreds of Web sites that will sell you capsules and powders of shark cartilage and claim cancer cures. Without a randomized, controlled trial, so-called cures are pure speculation. Until these hucksters show you the science, please don't show them your money.

Are there really advances? Yes, of course.

Advances in the treatment of cancer are agonizingly slow, have many false stops and starts, and lead even the most conscientious scientist down multiple dead ends. However, with persistence, tenacity, and a little good luck, some striking findings are now being developed and reported in the headlines.

Aggressive and often deadly forms of leukemia include chronic myeloid leukemia and acute lymphoblastic leukemia. About forty years ago, patients with chronic myeloid leukemia were discovered to have an unusual chromosome entitled the Philadelphia chromosome. This enzyme is detected in almost all cases of the leukemia and in a smaller proportion of patients with acute lymphoblastic leukemia. Several years ago, scientists published a fascinating study on the role of a chemical initially called ST1571, now called Gleevec. This medication specifically blocked or deactivated an enzyme called tyrosine kinase, which was present in the patients with these two forms of leukemia. The findings were striking in that more than half of these patients with each form of leukemia had remarkable benefits, and the side effects were quite manageable and tolerable. These findings suggested that there could be "targeted therapy" or "smart treatments" specifically honing in on a biochemical abnormality in the cancer cell.

These findings have now been extended to patients with other cancers, most notably an unusual form of tumor called gastrointestinal stromal tumors. Again, the results have been striking and the side effects relatively modest. In other words, in this case there is a "heat-seeking missile" that goes directly to the cancer cells, rather than a nonspecific treatment such as chemotherapy, which attacks all rapidly dividing cells both malignant and nonmalignant and causes a whole host of side effects (nausea, vomiting, risks of bleeding and infection).

Believe me, researchers are hunched over their microscopes conducting intense studies to determine the value of this type of medication in a variety of other cancers.

The lesson is that the tireless efforts of scientists in laboratories throughout the country, at some point in time, have the potential of providing the key to unlock the secret of cancer. We need to be realistic. It is not likely that one medication and the interruption of one enzyme will apply to all cancers, but the Gleevec story truly is a success story (but not an overnight success story) in which we can all take hope from the headlines.

My Thoughts . . .

Medicine is changing at a blistering pace. No one practitioner can know all there is to know on any one subject. But you can know everything you need to know about you. Whether you're in the doctor's office or a patient in a hospital, getting a new prescription, or having a regular checkup, it's critical for you to be your own best watchdog and advocate. The informed patient and family can better partner with their providers to get the best results as you journey down whatever path your medical history takes you.

When your search for medical knowledge takes you to mainstream media, understand the minefields and be skeptical about the headlines. Articles published in peer-reviewed medical journals are just that—communication within the scientific world exchanging ideas and findings. Sometimes this information becomes headline news when, in reality, it's not ready for prime time. The Internet allows even more users (not just medical personnel) to access medical information and journals that they never would have read in the past.

Opening this medical world is good if used and interpreted in context, but when laboratory findings among fourteen volunteers in Finland become headline news in Cedar Rapids, Iowa, the problems crop up in doctors' offices across the country. When science and the media give mixed signals, our patients get their hopes up, and we doctors are left to explain the cold, hard reality.

Part Three

ESSENTIAL STEPS TO
SURVIVING ANY DIAGNOSIS

10

What Do I Have?
What Should I Do? Why?

*There are some things you learn best
in calm and some in storm.*

—Willa Cather

As a practicing medical oncologist for almost thirty years, I have had the privilege of caring for thousands of patients and their families during the darkest days of their lives—and witnessed some of the most triumphant. During this time, I have made some observations about mistakes patients make (these are predictable, and you can avoid making them). I firmly believe that patients can (and *must*) be their own best advocate. And I have made some bedside observations about how best to cope with and improve your outcome from a dread disease—or any disease or condition, not just cancer.

You can view your medical decisions much like you might view critical business decisions. In fact, I advise you to create a board of directors (made up of your closest family and wisest friends). If you're the patient with a potentially life-threatening condition, make yourself chairman. Appoint a cabinet of advisers (this is your medical team). But remember, you are the one sitting at the head of that table. You're the final decision maker. You're in charge.

I hope you will use the following advice as a guide to drilling deeper into the questions people need to ask when they become patients. I urge you to work with your medical-care providers to receive the thoughtful, respectful and learned answers—and care—you deserve.

Know Your Diagnosis

First, you need to know what's going on with you—that's your diagnosis. If it's a broken arm, a brain tumor, heart attack, stroke, diabetes, lupus, or any other condition or disease, minor or major, you need to know what's happening, so you can access information about the problem on your own and recover from it. Even better, if you can see the enemy, you can fight it. So insist on seeing your x-rays, lab results, CT scans, mammograms, bone scans and MRIs.

Acknowledge the seriousness of your diagnosis. This involves knowing the name of the cancer under the microscope, the size and grade of the cancer, and whether or not this is viewed as a slow-growing or an aggressive process. You need to know if you have type 1 or type 2 diabetes, what kind of heart attack you have had and how much heart damage you may have sustained, and whether your stroke was caused by a blockage or bleeding. Without knowing the details about your condition, you cannot access information about the problem on your own and make informed decisions about your treatment.

My best advice

Bring along a family member or friend (someone from your "medical" board of directors) who can think clearly and act as your advocate by asking questions and writing down the doctors' responses. Why? Because most patients retain very little information when their circuits are overloaded from being presented with a serious diagnosis.

Be in Charge

Next, create an equal partnership between you and your primary-care physician or specialist. Don't give up or just go along with medical decisions made by someone else. Ask your family and friends for support, but do not proceed with treatment just because they think it is the "right" thing to do. You are all allied against a common foe (your disease) with hopes of achieving one of three goals: a cure, quality time or decreased symptoms.

You and your doctor have equal responsibility for the outcome, but you as an empowered patient (or a knowledgeable family member acting on your behalf if you are unable) will make the ultimate decisions about your treatment. Gone are the days when families and doctors conspired to keep the true diagnosis of a dread disease from the patient to spare them the fear of the outcome.

Make certain that you get copies of letters from your specialist to your primary doctor. Keep your operative and pathology reports, especially if you plan to seek a second opinion. Your medical records are your property, but be aware that you may not understand all the techno-speak, and that can cause lots of anguish if you don't understand what the medical terms mean.

Keep in mind that you, the patient (or you as the advocate for your parent or spouse or child or friend), need to be appropriately assertive in treatment decisions. Speak up. Be involved. It's your life.

Don't ask the doctor what he or she would do in similar circumstances. It's tempting to go along with the doctor who says, "Well, if you were my mother . . ." or "I'd advise my golfing buddy . . ." They are not you.

When my patients ask what I would do, I explain that what may be right for me may not be okay for the patient sitting in front of me under the same circumstances. Here's an example. I know the risks of chemotherapy. If the chance of benefit is low, and if side effects are high, I may not elect treatment. But some patients will grasp at any remedy, even if the odds of benefit are one in a thousand. I'd opt for quality time. Some patients, on the other hand, play the odds.

My best advice

Is it obvious by now that I want patients to be in charge?

Knowledge Is Powerful Medicine

At all times, be active and appropriately assertive. You're in a foreign environment in your new role as patient. You don't know the language or how the game is played. But you can learn, just as you may have learned about the financial world to invest in the stock market or learned the ins and outs of buying and selling on eBay. Knowing the language of medicine will help you talk effectively with the medical specialists holding your future.

I admire the parents who become experts practically overnight when their child has a devastatingly gloomy diagnosis. One couple not only became experts in a very rare condition called RRP when their daughter was diagnosed, they formed a nonprofit foundation to support research, raised funds for researchers in this area, set up family and patient support groups, and even published medical papers with the few experts who truly know this life-threatening condition. Do these nonmedical people know about this condition? Yes, more than most professionals. Where did they learn about RRP? By reading everything they could in medical libraries and online at medical-library sites such as PubMed, by networking with patients and their families, and by asking questions of professionals who work with this disease. Plug into like-minded support groups, if appropriate for you.

You don't have to become a world expert, but you need to understand your condition before you can make decisions. Use your newfound knowledge when talking with your doctor. Yet if you don't understand what the doctor is saying, ask and insist on an answer you can grasp.

Many of my colleagues and I are seeing an increasing proportion of patients who are bringing information downloaded from the Internet to the bedside and the clinic. On occasion, this information can produce an adversarial, confrontational environment rather than a mutually respectful consultation with an easy exchange of information.

Interestingly, in my own experience it is family members and friends who typically come to the clinic armed with online information. In general, patients may be too ill or frightened to seek out information and therefore rely on the input of friends and family. This is certainly normal and appropriate, but ultimately, the patient is in the driver's seat and makes the decision about his or her own health and welfare.

Caution: Be careful of a well-meaning friend who dumps onto your lap a pile of wacko articles obtained from untrustworthy Web sites. They're usually worthless. Be leery of the friend who offers to sell you vitamins or supplements to "cure" you, even if the friend is from your church or bridge club.

The emergence of the Internet has provided us all with access to tens of thousands of Web sites specifically focusing on health issues. The total number of pages on the Internet has surpassed 1 billion, compared to a third as many pages just a few years ago. The information on the Internet can be your best ally or your worst enemy. Make it your ally, by using the information from trusted medical sources to make yourself the smartest patient your doctor has ever treated. Be wary of sites sponsored by companies hoping to sell you a product. Access sites from universities, the federal government and nationally known nonprofit health organizations. If you do not know how to use this tool, friends and family can surely help.

But, sadly, some of the information on the Internet is flat-out wrong, dangerous and unreliable. Do you really think if you authorize $29.95 by credit card to *cancercures-R-US.com,* you will find what others have never found? You need to be careful. If a program sounds too good to be true, it is.

The hallmarks of a credible Web site are credentials. Well-known universities and medical centers are a sure bet. These sites will have few advertisements, if any, and won't try to lure you to their centers for treatment.

Web sites in which "doctors" give specific advice can be appealing but dangerous. Check out these so-called cyber docs or alternative practitioners with an independent source. You can look up the backgrounds of medical professionals on various sites on the Internet (a list is provided in the back of this book). You're looking for medical degrees from places you've heard of to establish their credibility, not a questionable "offshore" diploma or medical degree by mail order. Even dogs can get degrees from universities advertising their credentialing programs on banner ads.

Comparing your case with that of a friend, neighbor or colleague is unwise. Patients cannot be expected to understand the subtleties and nuances of each individual's case. To compare your situation with that of a neighbor with the "same cancer" or "same stroke" or "same heart attack" can be risky, dangerous and cause lots of sleepless nights. That's like comparing legal cases or financial portfolios. Each case is unique.

The Internet is transforming civilization in general and the practice of medicine in particular unlike any other technology in the history of the world. It has taken the telephone approximately one hundred years to connect us as a global communication family. The Internet has performed the same feat in less than one hundred months.

The numbers are staggering. Some experts estimate that within five years, a billion individuals will be on the Internet. Think about it. That's one out of every six people on the planet.

And what does this mean for the patient and the family? Let me use a primitive example of myself as an amateur financial analyst.

Because of powerful search engines and financial sites sponsored by companies, I now have access to obscure information that was previously available only to stockbrokers and financial analysts. Now let me be perfectly clear. I may not have the sophistication of some of the experts, but I can get a very clear sense of market trends, prudent investment strategies, and the kinds of ideas that are completely off-base and irresponsible. In a sense, the playing field has been leveled. The knowledge gap between me as the consumer and the financial professional has been narrowed because of the Internet. I'm able to at least know the questions to ask and can avoid some mine fields as I pilot my financial future in a murky and uncharted arena.

Now the same thought process applies to the patient. Health information and medically related topics are among the most sought-after information on the Internet. With powerful search engines such as Yahoo, Lycos, Alta Vista, Google and others, even the completely computer-illiterate individual can type in a few key phrases of the diagnosis and have instant access to the world's literature on their desktop. So how do the patient and family know which is reliable and which is downright dangerous?

Some general guidelines are worth mentioning:

- A responsible site is sponsored by a national medical organization, such as the American Heart Association, the American Cancer Society or the Academy of Family Practitioners.
- Sites that promote the philosophy and ideas of a single celebrity/scientist/physician may be factual but might also be tainted by commercial interests.
- Be leery of sites that are sponsored by a single corporation, especially a pharmaceutical firm. Many are honorable and do an excellent job, but commercial interests may cloud judgment and reasoning.
- Sites sponsored by major universities and medical centers typically

have reliable information. However, some medical centers are for-profit, so you must be wary of their attempts to lure patients into their practices.

- If the corners of a site are littered with advertisements popping up for fancy medical devices and medications, watch out, you might be enticed hook, line and wallet.

Now what do you do with reliable information once you've schooled yourself? While I may have access to financial information and financial data, I do not have financial wisdom, and that's where I need the input of the professional. So it is with the patient.

My best advice

Learn the language of your illness or condition. Stick with the Web sites operated by nationally known interest groups and medical centers. You'll also find the government sites particularly thorough and reliable, as are sites run by health-serving organizations, such as the American Cancer Society, American Lung Association, American Diabetes Association, Crohn's and Colitis Foundation of America, American Heart Association, and many others. Start your search at a major health portal. To start at a major search engine such as Google or Yahoo would be like stepping into uncharted territory. The final section of this book contains a helpful listing of Web sites and health portals.

Explore Your Treatment Options

Your doctor will lay out your options, but the buck stops with you. It's your decision which path you pursue. Ask the pros and cons of medication, surgery, diet and further sophisticated testing. Make sure you know the goal of treatment. Decide what you are "buying" with each option or combination of options. You could be buying poor quality of life after a highly toxic treatment to live a little longer instead of opting for peaceful quality family time. You can do nothing: One often-overlooked option is to accept *no* treatment, especially for certain types of cancers.

Ask your doctor these questions to help you make your decisions:

- **Is this disease curable or controllable or confinable?** Don't accept a response of "we don't know." Doctors do know certain scenarios based on the experiences of similar groups of patients with the same type of disease. Each person's disease is different, but doctors can get in the ballpark.
- **What are my chances of getting improvement from this treatment?** If you aren't satisfied with the response, seek a second opinion from another medical center specializing in the condition you have. It's your right, and it's your future. Ask your doctor for an immediate referral. Some doctors may even sense your discomfort about the treatment plan and offer to set up a second opinion. One second opinion—no more than two—should give you enough information to make a decision. Don't waste your time waiting in airports and medical offices shopping for an opinion you like.
- **Am I eligible for any experimental treatments?** Ask if you can take part in clinical trials but be certain to understand the difference between Phase 1 and Phase 2 trials. Phase 1 studies assess new agents. The programs are designed to find the best dose of the medication. Phase 2 agents have some promise but rarely offer a cure. Beware of going to a foreign land for the "cure." If we, as the greatest country for medical progress, do not have the answer, do you really think a third-world country has some hidden secret potion?

My best advice

Get the big picture and then make your treatment decision.

Ask for a Second Opinion

Don't be shy. Recognize the importance of a second opinion. No single institution and no single physician or health-care provider can have complete information about every condition. As professionals, they should not be offended if you want to seek a second opinion. This is a common practice in medicine today.

If a major medical center or university has a particular expertise in your disease, it certainly makes good sense to seek a second opinion there. Almost never will the local physician be offended, and if he or she is, that is even more reason to seek another opinion. Support groups in the city where the medical center is located or bona fide groups on the Internet can provide names of local experts. Call on one with your doctor's support.

But be realistic and spend your time profitably. To fly all over the country to get seventeen different opinions from a variety of medical centers is bewildering, diffusing and enormously expensive—not only in terms of dollars and cents but also in terms of wasted time. One or possibly two confirmatory opinions at the most are more than adequate to provide some reasonable directions for treatment. Avoid the paralysis of analysis. At some point, just do it: Follow treatment recommendations or not.

Once you commit to a course of action, be an active patient and partner in your treatment. Know your medication and previous treatment. It is astonishing that patients tell me they take "a little yellow pill and a little white pill" and have no understanding about the name of the medications, who prescribed them or why. This is not a good practice. Likewise, know dosages, schedules and the names of previous drugs you have taken. This will help the doctors provide the best care during a very difficult situation. Keep a log or diary to help you remember what was said and recommended and why.

My best advice

When you're not satisfied with your diagnosis, treatment or progress, you'll want to get a second opinion.

Take Time to Take Your Best Shot

Any serious diagnosis is devastating and paralyzing. The very words, "You have cancer," or "Your child has muscular dystrophy," overwhelm our senses of judgment and reasoning. So take time to think about your course of action before you rush to treatment.

With many conditions, the signs and symptoms may have been present for a long time, not just since yesterday. Therefore, there usually is no real urgency to rush into treatment within a day or two of diagnosis (stroke and heart attacks are exceptions where life-saving treatment must be started within hours). Keep in mind that many treatment options cannot be reversed. For example, removal of a breast or prostate is a major life-altering event.

Have some understanding of the natural history of your disease. Ask your doctor to explain the typical track record and progression. As with most situations in life, your first shot is the best. If the first-string team is not winning, what chance does the second-string have? If the first kind of treatment does not work, the patient usually is weaker and sicker, making the success of the second treatment low. Not zero. But low.

My best advice

Gather all the information and opinions and then make informed decisions to take your best shot.

Set Up Your Support System and Keep Everyone Thinking Positively

Social connectedness is one of the biggest factors in explaining why some patients do better with serious illness than others. Well-controlled studies have shown that the support of family, friends and even pets lifts spirits mentally and boosts immune systems physically [for more on this, please see chapter 12]. Families need to be supportive of the patient's decisions—no matter what those decisions are.

My best advice

Tap into your network. Assemble your board of directors and discuss the options for care, treatment, recovery and rehabilitation. Remember who's chairing the meeting: *you*.

Do Not Second-Guess
Your Health-Care Decisions

Don't look back. Plan ahead. Trust your instincts on your treatment and maintain a comfort level with your care-providing team. If you don't think someone is acting in your best interest, get someone who is.

On Monday morning, everyone is an expert quarterback. This also applies to picking winning stocks. Energies need to be focused on today and not on past events. To ruminate over diagnostic tests that should have been done or treatments that were not effective simply takes energy away from the task at hand. Focus on relationships, priorities and the to-do list. What is important becomes obvious: family and friends, not all the other "stuff" that distracts us.

My best advice

Carpe diem: "Seize the day." Savor each opportunity. After all, today is really all that any of us has.

Life Is a Full-Time Job—Set Priorities

Don't let the rest of your life unravel while you deal with treatment. Life when you're healthy is a full-time job. Be realistic when you're operating at less than 100 percent. Cut back. Slow down and smell the roses.

Recognize that there is no such thing as Superman or Superwoman. Fighting a disease, too, is a full-time job. It is foolish to think that you can deal with the rigors of certain treatments, such as chemotherapy or physical rehabilitation, maintain a business or an active work life, and run a household without some sort of help.

Nobody can go it alone, and now is the time to reach out and seek the help you need from friends and neighbors. Acknowledge the importance of a support system. A friend or confidante can be an anchor during stormy times. Don't ignore the resources of your religious group, if you have one.

Acknowledge your limitations. As a result of treatment, your energy, vitality and focus may well diminish. It is not reasonable to continue to work fifty hours a week, reshingle the roof and put on a dinner party for the country club crowd, all while dealing with serious side effects or recovery challenges. Prioritize, make lists, acknowledge that there are limitations to your stamina. Do not hesitate to tell people that you need rest and time alone.

Take charge of your time. If you work sixty hours a week, understand that you may not have the energy to keep up that pace during treatment and recovery, so do what's most important in the first half of your day. It's up to you to decide what's most important and how to spend your time profitably.

My best advice

Time will take on new meaning. Make the most of it.

My Thoughts . . .

When faced with an alarming diagnosis, many people don't know what to do, or what to do first. I've set out the essential steps to surviving any diagnosis.

Some of my patients face grim decisions about equally bleak futures. One thought that keeps me going is that "hope is a presence that erases the limitations on possibilities for the future." The absence of hope eliminates any possibilities. With my patients, we never give up hope.

Whatever you face, I advise you to be appropriately optimistic, appropriately proactive and appropriately realistic. Please recognize that there is a window of uncertainty as the journey of life unfolds.

We in medicine must embrace life's uncertainties because we don't have all the answers.

The Search for Health, Peace and Serenity in Complementary Medicine

Much of your pain is the bitter potion
by which the physician within you heals your sick self.

—Kahlil Gibran

Many people, when grasping for help with a life-threatening illness, give up on scientifically proven, mainstream medical care and believe if they go to Greece or the Bahamas or Mexico they will find some magic cure—usually for cancer.

I've had personal experiences when patients on this quest would die in a foreign hospital—thousands of miles from home. If that wasn't tragic enough, before the family could leave the local motel to rush to their loved one's bedside, the body of the deceased was stripped, rings were taken from it and exorbitant fees were then extorted from the patient's family to return the body to the United States.

That's alternative medicine at its worst.

When faced with a life-threatening illness, especially one charged with a potentially fatal verdict, it is reasonable and understandable that patients will seek virtually every possible option to come to grips with their illness.

Here we are at the dawn of the twenty-first century with the greatest marvels in the history of medicine, the most advanced diagnostic armamentarium, the finest surgeons and the greatest hospitals in the world. Yet there is a nagging dissatisfaction with the medical-care delivery system. An element of disillusionment exists. But there are definitely no miracle cures in Timbuktu.

What I hear every day in the clinic goes something like this: "If we can put a man on the moon, we can certainly cure cancer." But here is the problem. We have long understood the physics, the mechanics and the engineering principles of launching a satellite to a distant galaxy. However, for most cancers right here on our planet, we do not have the foggiest notion of why one cell goes haywire, becomes bizarre, spreads and ultimately takes away a person's life. Patients are frustrated, families are disillusioned and seek out alternative or complementary therapies in their search for that "something else."

What's Your Alternative?

Although firm figures are not always available, many experts have suggested that at least 70 percent of patients—and more—use techniques and interventions that do not fall under the traditional umbrella of usual and customary medical practices. I'm talking about complementary and alternative medicine, as defined by the government's National Center for Complementary and Alternative Medicine:

- **Alternative medical systems:** Truly alternative forms of medicine would be homeopathic and naturopathic medicine and traditional Chinese medicine and Ayurveda.
  - Homeopathic practitioners believe that "like cures like." They administer small, highly diluted medicinal substances to cure symptoms, when the same substances at higher doses would actually cause those symptoms.
  - With naturopathic medicine, practitioners work with natural healing forces within the body. Such practices may include diet, massage and acupuncture to promote healing and better health.
  - Traditional Chinese medicine (TCM) targets the body's life force, or *qi,* through diet, massage, herbs and acupuncture.

—Ayurveda comes to us from India and marshals the mind, body and spirit in disease prevention and treatment.

- **Mind–body interventions:** We'll discuss the mind–body connection further, but techniques, such as patient support groups and cognitive behavioral therapy, once thought to be a little "out there," have become quite mainstream. True mind–body techniques include meditation, prayer, mental healing, and creative uses of art, music and dance.

- **Biologically based therapies:** Substances found in nature such as herbs, foods and vitamins—globally thought of as dietary supplements—fall into this category. Not everything found in nature is therapeutic, of course, and just because something is called "natural" doesn't make it safe. Lard, for example, is quite natural, but is hardly safe.

- **Manipulative and body-based methods:** Chiropractors manipulate muscles, joints and tendons, and these practitioners can relieve tension and pain, but they cannot cure cancer. Many well-trained chiropractors today recognize their limitations and can provide relief for some people, typically working in concert with the traditional medical practitioner.

- **Energy therapies:** Some people think that energy fields surround and penetrate the human body, although this has not been scientifically proven. Practitioners of biofield therapies such as qi gong, Reiki and therapeutic touch say they manipulate the energy fields by applying pressure or manipulating the body using their hands. A more intense form of this type of therapy involves electromagnetic fields— also not proven.

These products and techniques generally are not part of the mainstream, Western medical practice in doctors' offices and hospitals. Some alternative practices have been tried and rejected, and perhaps some of those just mentioned will move more into acceptance or fall out of favor. Let's look at past practices:

- At one time, there was tremendous enthusiasm for the visualization technique in which you would sit in a quiet room and envision your immune cells gobbling up cancer cells. Unfortunately, this technique has not withstood the test of time.

- Several years later, great interest was given to specific dietary regimens such as the macrobiotic diet, which was touted as a cancer cure. Unfortunately, brown rice is not the answer.

- Treatments called the Gerson Program as well as immuno-augmentative therapy have been popularized by a doctor in the Bahamas. These achieved great popularity but have never been proven to be of reasonable benefit. In fact, some of these practices might be unsafe because they restrict vital nutrients and certain minerals.

- Some practitioners advocated enemas with coffee and other types of interventions, which are not only useless, but downright dangerous. They opened clinics outside the United States. They made considerable sums of money and offered hope but with a sizable price tag. None of these treatments has ever withstood the scrutiny of appropriate clinical study.

- We are now into the era of megadose vitamin supplements, and likewise these have not consistently been a benefit.

The general terminology is to focus on the concept of *complementary* rather than the word *alternative*. Complementary suggests that these are adjuncts, these are programs in addition to, rather than substituting for, traditional medicine. I don't use the term *holistic;* no one has really pinned down a definition for it.

Complementary medicine or integrative medicine, on the other hand, combines mainstream medical therapies with alternative practices that have proven safety and effectiveness. Let me give you an example. Programs involving meditation, yoga and prayerful reflection can have a very positive impact on individuals struggling with chronic pain. These types of activities can be marshaled in conjunction with traditional pain programs using codeine and morphine. Therefore, the distinction is made between *alternative* and the preferable designation as *complementary.*

It is important that your primary health-care providers understand that you are participating in any type of complementary program. Research from Harvard's Center for Alternative Medical Research and Education (yes, mainstream medical schools are taking complementary medicine seriously) is revealing regarding the habits of those seeking alternative treatments.

- Most people who saw a medical doctor and used some sort of alternative practice felt the combination of the two was better than either one alone.

- Most people visit their primary-care physician before seeing an alternative practitioner. But those seeing both types of caregivers felt equal confidence in their providers' abilities—not necessarily less confidence in modern medical practice.

- Among those who saw an alternative practitioner and a medical doctor, up to 72 percent did not disclose that they'd visited an alternative practitioner when talking to the medical doctor. They felt it wasn't important for the medical doctor to know, or the doctor never asked, or it was none of the doctor's business, they responded. A few felt their doctor might disapprove or discourage use of alternative medicine.

And this is where the problem lies. Sometimes serious interactions can occur between antibiotics, blood-thinning medications and herbal remedies. There's also another factor of which we need to be mindful. Patients are buying alternative medications on the Internet and at shopping malls.

When you buy an antibiotic or antidepressant or a heart medication, you can be reasonably certain that safeguards of purity and manufacturing standards have been followed. This is not always the case when you buy an over-the-counter nutritional supplement, herbal or vitamin—even at the corner drugstore. So you need to be reasonable and share this information with all your health-care providers—alternative and otherwise.

Worthless or Worthwhile—How Can We Tell?

The notion of complementary or alternative therapies generally refers to interventions that are not uniformly embraced by the rank and file of traditional medical practitioners. Now does this mean these treatments are worthless? Certainly not. Now you're waiting for the other shoe to drop. With proper study, we can find out whether a mainstream treatment is worthwhile or worthless. And the same scientific inquiry can be used to examine alternative therapies. Here are two examples:

To C or not to C

Dr. Linus Pauling is the only person in the world to have won three Nobel Prizes. So when he speaks, the world listens. When Dr. Pauling began touting the value of high doses of vitamin C to treat cancer (he said he himself took megadoses every day), many people began adding vitamin C to their daily routines.

Many of the more skeptical medical critics said Dr. Pauling's studies were flawed. His patients who received vitamin C were compared with patient records obtained from a hospital in Scotland. This technique is called historical review and is no longer accepted as a scientific standard to assess the benefit of therapy. Needless to say, I myself was among the skeptics.

We at Mayo Clinic performed a prospective, randomized clinical trial to address this issue. The technique of our study represented the gold standard of assessing a therapy. The patients in our study had far-advanced cancer and were rigorously analyzed by a team of statisticians.

Bottom line: There was no advantage for the patients who received vitamin C in the management of advanced cancer. Our results were published in *The New England Journal of Medicine*—one of the most prestigious and rigorously reviewed medical journals in the world.

Since then, in general, high doses of vitamin C have somewhat fallen by the wayside and are no longer on the radar screen of most cancer patients. At least, not for long.

We were strongly criticized by Dr. Pauling and his colleagues for the way we performed our study. Nevertheless, we stood our ground, and our findings (which followed rigorous scientific methods) could not show benefit for vitamin C for patients with advanced cancer.

We then performed a second study of individuals who had advanced cancer, but the cancer had been removed surgically. For example, someone might have had a cancer arising from the colon and rectum, which spread into the liver. The cancer in the liver was removed. Though the patients were "disease-free," they were at very high risk for a recurrence of the same cancer. These patients were generally healthier than those who had far-advanced cancer in the earlier study. We again embarked upon a trial in which patients were given either a placebo (pills with no medication in them) or a high dose of vitamin C. In the findings, once again, we could see no benefit whatsoever from the vitamin C.

Now let's take this issue one step further. Is it possible that if vitamin C is taken throughout one's life that it would act as a preventive medication and block the development of cancer? The answers are unclear. Theoretically, maybe yes. But at the present time, there is no convincing or compelling evidence that vitamin C as a preventive intervention will avoid the development of cancer down the road.

This is the pits

Laetrile is a chemical extracted from apricot pits. It was touted as the answer to the cancer problem. A miracle cure. In the 1980s, an entire underground economy grew out of bootlegging laetrile from various parts of the world, including Mexico. Like drug smugglers, these greedy "drug" dealers and well-meaning family members would do just about anything and pay any price to get laetrile for cancer patients.

Under the direction of Charles Moertel, M.D., who had been the Chair of the Comprehensive Cancer Center at Mayo Clinic, researchers conducted a scientifically valid, meticulously detailed study and clinical trials. Again, no benefit from laetrile. And its use dropped off.

The Placebo Effect—Sleight of Mind?

Perhaps one explanation for the value of some of these supplements and techniques (bogus or otherwise) is the "placebo effect." In other words, if you have a strong belief system that a certain intervention or a certain medication will work, it is possible that that belief will trigger the production of immune-related agents—chemicals deep within the brain that resemble opium. This might account for the so-called "runner's high" and the ability of individuals when under stress to carry on in the face of broken bones and penetrating injuries.

There are a variety of brain chemicals called endorphins, which probably make us less aware of pain and, at least on a short-term basis, can increase stamina and a sense of well-being. In other words, if we strongly believe in the value of an intervention, it might be of some benefit, at least in the short-term.

Many of us may dimly remember a history lecture that included a discussion about the mind–body connection. The first civilization to promote this concept gave birth to Socrates and Aristotle. The Greeks have brought many gifts into the world, and one of these was the concept that we cannot separate the mind and the body. What affects one, affects the other. Any sort of separation of these two phenomena is artificial. What we think, we become. Our language creates our reality.

Would you like a demonstration of the mind–body connection? Close your eyes and visualize a juicy lemon. See it. Feel it. Smell its freshness. Now cut open your lemon and squeeze the juice into a glass.

At what point did your mouth begin watering? Or your lips pucker? This wasn't a response you needed to think about. It just happened. Where did your mind end and your bodily function begin? This is the mind–body interface.

Through similar self-imagery and mindful meditative thought, you can even lower your blood pressure, calm your brain waves and control your heart rate.

Let me tell you a story. The patient was a woman in her early sixties. She had far-advanced colon cancer with extensive involvement of the liver. The capsule of the liver is much like the covering of a football in terms of texture and thickness. It is filled with delicate nerve endings that are incredibly sensitive to pain caused by the liver expanding from the growth of the cancer. This patient was admitted to the hospital with severe pain.

She made a very clear statement to each of us on rounds one morning: "If I were a dog, you'd shoot me. If I were a horse, you would put me down. Please end this misery." We marshaled the very best narcotic regimen that medicine can bring to the bedside. We brought to the patient the most sophisticated computer-driven technology to meticulously deliver doses of pain-numbing medicines. Our results were increasingly futile over the patient's first hospital days.

A member of the medical team asked during a morning visit, "Do you have a church affiliation or a minister who might be of some help?"

Almost miraculously, our patient's demeanor changed, and she agreed to visit with one of our chaplains. And then her story unfolded. It was a tale of betrayal, resentment and bitterness about a devastating blow she and her husband had endured from an uncaring corporate giant. Once she found a kind listener, she could verbalize her anger at the unfairness of life. At that point, we were able to dramatically decrease the doses of morphine, and she was discharged virtually pain-free.

The lesson is clear. This is not rocket science—or even medical science. We can drip in all sorts of narcotic cocktails to relieve the patient's pain. However, if we do not acknowledge that many of us have pain in the soul and if that pain is not addressed and acknowledged, it is highly unlikely that all the morphine in the world will bring the patients the peace and serenity they so desperately need.

Placebo? Or mind and body at work? Does it matter as long as the patient finds help, hope and healing? We need them all in our arsenal.

The Irony of Herbs and Vitamins

I'm supportive when patients want to try herbal remedies. I'm understanding about vitamins. But I try to point out the potential problems in taking any of these dietary supplements—they're not regulated, they could contain a host of contaminants. I try to discourage patients from wasting a lot of money and creating what some colleagues call "expensive urine" (because what your body does not use, you excrete).

Although experts say most herbs are safe when taken as directed, a recent series of FDA warnings and product recalls underscores the fact that these products are not tested, inspected or given a seal of approval—by anybody. The Dietary Supplement Health and Education Act (DSHEA), passed in 1994, does not require manufacturers of herbs and other dietary supplements to prove that their products are safe or effective before they hit the shelves. Manufacturers can make general health claims on their labels, without any regulation about what they say.

You are unprotected when you buy herbals. In fact, a professor at Duke University Medical Center said, "You know more about what is in a bag of Doritos than what's in an herbal product touted to treat and prevent disease." There's no guarantee these products are safe or effective.

Death, liver damage, seizure, heart attack and stroke have all occurred as a result of consumers using a small number of herbal products, according to FDA alerts and advisories, most recently on ephedra (ma huang) and St. John's wort. Such adverse events can be caused by herbal products interacting with other medicines, allergies, impurities, and when taken in dangerously high doses.

Like many of the known risks of herbal medicines, these hazards were revealed after the products went on the market. In a sense, you are the laboratory test animal.

Still attached to your herbal of choice? Certainly hedge your bets and don't create dangerous interactions. Be aware that herbals and prescription medications may not mix well. Discuss everything you take with your doctor. Bring the bottle so you can examine the labeling together. Some things just shouldn't be taken in combination. Let me give you some examples:

- **Echinacea:** This herbal stimulates the immune system. That's why people often take it to avoid colds, but it can be a problem for people who take medications such as prednisone or corticosteroids or organ transplant drugs to decrease the activity of their immune system. Avoid it if you use alcohol because echinacea can cause liver problems in some people already prone to liver damage.
- **Garlic:** Garlic contains bacteria-fighting properties that can slow blood from clotting, so if you take blood thinners such as aspirin, warfarin or other anticoagulants, you may be at risk for bleeding. Garlic can even change the results of your blood-clotting tests. People who take arthritis pain medications also may be at risk for bruising if taking garlic. And garlic may increase the effect of blood sugar–lowering drugs for those who take diabetes medications. Garlic cooked in foods becomes inactivated because of the heat and is okay. Interactions can occur with fresh garlic and concentrated supplements.
- **Ginseng:** Some people take ginseng to increase their resistance to stress, anemia, depression and other chronic illness. Avoid ginseng if you take blood thinners including aspirin and warfarin because it may interfere with their ability to work. Ginseng also lowers blood sugar in people who take medicine for diabetes.
- **Gingko biloba:** This extract is often taken for circulatory problems and memory enhancement. It inhibits the blood's ability to form clots, so if taken with blood thinners, even aspirin or vitamin E, you may experience bleeding. Anyone taking thiazide (water pills) may experience an increase in blood pressure.
- **St. John's wort:** Taken for mild depression, this herbal can increase the liver's ability to remove other medications so they become less effective. When used in combination with other antidepressants such as Prozac, the interaction can cause an excessive antidepressant effect. St. John's wort also can make some birth control pills less effective. And I advise against it for anyone undergoing chemotherapy.
- **Valerian:** An herbal used to calm nervousness is mildly sedating. When combined with a prescription drug for the same purpose, or with alcohol, the effects add up and can cause confusion and extreme tiredness.

But what about regular old vitamins? There has been renewed interest in the past decade in antioxidant vitamins such as vitamins C and E and dietary supplements such as selenium and zinc. The compelling scientific evidence supporting the value of these substances is simply not there. Not yet.

But should you be discouraged from taking them? It's best that you discuss your interest with your doctor so that you each understand the pros, cons, risks and options of taking any supplements or vitamins. I cannot imagine most doctors having great resistance to their patients taking vitamins if well informed.

A little vitamin C as part of a multivitamin falls in the category of "won't hurt." But megadoses of vitamin C, as espoused by Dr. Linus Pauling, can be toxic. That's the difference.

A great amount of research has been done involving antioxidants. We're not exactly sure how they work, or if they work at all. Now a brief word about biochemistry.

There is some evidence that, as we age, the body produces chemicals called "free radicals." These free radicals, in some circumstances, can ignite or start the growth of cancer, and these chemicals might have something to do with the development of heart disease. If you can block the development of free radicals by medication called antioxidants, there is the hope that the cancer may not occur or that heart disease might not occur, or so goes the thinking.

Again, there is a tremendous gap between the research in the laboratory and the practical application of this research when you're looking at a shelf of vitamins and wondering if you need to take them. In general, antioxidants obtained from what we eat (in fruits and vegetables) are probably better than the antioxidants obtained in a tablet form you buy at the drugstore. At one time, some thought vitamin E, for example, would be helpful against heart disease, but that issue is still controversial. Likewise, the role of antioxidants as a way to prevent cancer, although theoretically appealing, has not withstood the scrutiny of rigorously conducted clinical trials.

Open Your Mouth and Say "Om"

Health is the greatest gift, contentment the greatest wealth, faithfulness the best relationship.

—Buddha

Scientists are not quite certain how meditation works, but perhaps we can gain some insight from the work of Harvard's Herbert Benson, M.D., who initially wrote about the relaxation response. Dr. Benson's work has shown that images of a quiet stream or a flower-laden forest can lower blood pressure, lower pulse and have tremendous benefits for those with coronary artery disease.

Picturing serenity, achieving bliss in your mind's eye—this is the very basis of human pursuits. Through mental imagery, transcendental or Kundalini meditation and other meditation techniques, prayer and other types of cerebral activities, people fight disease. Whether or not these techniques prolong life is unclear, but they certainly enhance the quality of life and empower patients in this most difficult of all of life's journeys.

Now this brings us to the issue of stress. There is a general conception that stress somehow causes disease—from the common cold to cancer. However, few credible studies would fully support this statement. We do know, for example, that stress is a major factor in coronary artery disease (heart attacks), but the same statement cannot be said for cancer. But how can we deal with stress?

The meditation program called mindfulness-based stress reduction has been developed for patients with chronic illnesses and conditions, such as anxiety/panic disorder, asthma and allergies, cancer, depression, gastrointestinal problems, high blood pressure, chronic pain, sleep disorders, and stress. Researchers reporting on the technique say that nearly all participants in the study were continuing their meditative practices a year after the initial eight-week program. The training helped these patients cope with illness and stress. They were able to learn deep-breathing techniques to reduce body tension and increase mental clarity. Overall, they simply felt better and were better able to cope with their illnesses.

Meditation techniques are not a secret. Nor are they difficult to learn. You can find worthy programs taught through wellness and fitness centers, at universities, in hospital programs and at YMCAs. Some yoga programs incorporate meditation in the practice.

The meditation or yoga mantra—a word you repeat silently to trigger the relaxation response described by Dr. Benson at Harvard—can be powerful. Similar to prayer, the mantra can create measurable beneficial effects in your body. A study in Italy recorded the breathing rates of adults who either recited the rosary prayer or their yoga mantra. Both the mantra and the Ave Maria slowed breathing in the test subjects, improved their concentration, and induced calm and a feeling of well-being.

And then there is the power of prayer.

One of the first efforts to study the effects of complementary medicine practices was conducted at Duke University Medical Center with cardiac patients who required coronary stenting (a heart procedure to prop open the arteries).

Patients who received complementary interventions in addition to the stenting appeared to do better than those who simply had the operation. All patients received the stenting, but smaller groups of these patients also received one of four interventions: guided imagery, stress relaxation, healing touch or intercessory prayer (prayer groups of varying denominations around the world were given the name, age and illness of the patient assigned to them and prayed for the patients). Patients did not know whether they were being prayed for or whether they were receiving standard therapy without the prayer intervention.

Those receiving any of the four complementary interventions had lower absolute complication rates and fewer problems after surgery during hospitalization. Researchers suggest that the interventions helped patients feel more calm, which helps in the recovery process. Those assigned to receive prayer appeared to fare even better than those receiving the other types of complementary treatments and better than the control group. The results of this pilot study were so intriguing that a similar but larger study is ongoing at nine medical centers across the country.

My personal retreat

For the past fifteen years, I have dropped out of life for three days, typically in April, to go to Demontreville. This is a beautiful estate just east of St. Paul, Minnesota. On the grounds are a modest chapel, a communal eating area and five Dutch colonial–type homes, each of which can comfortably house seventy men.

This program has been in place for at least fifty years. There is a waiting list to participate in this retreat, which is held fifty-one weeks every year. The tone of the retreat follows the philosophy of St. Ignatius Loyola, the founder of the Jesuits. He believed that only with true quiet meditation and introspective reflection could one truly understand and tackle the great mysteries of life.

Typically a Jesuit retreat master will deliver two or three very brief homilies throughout each day. These last no more than ten or fifteen minutes and are then followed by one or two hours of reflection. The grounds are beautiful and are conducive to trying to sort out who we are and what our purpose in life really is. Overall there is a Catholic flavor to the program in terms of rituals, the Mass and the rosary. Yet many in attendance are non-Catholics. We are each in the same boat. The issues with which we struggle are clearly universal and apply to each one of us.

As a compulsive note taker, I quote faithfully and write down some of the key issues. Let me share with you what I wrote down following one recent retreat.

- **Don't worry—too much.** Scriptures tell us that if you worry too much, you may not go the distance in life and that no one ever added an inch to his or her life by worrying. It's also not good for your heart. Sacred scriptures and writings from a variety of traditions are a great source in comforting patients and sustaining them in these difficult times—and also their doctors.
- **Solitude is crucial for survival.** A patient with a life-challenging illness may become bombarded by advice and many times needs to be alone. This is especially challenging for the well-educated or socially prominent person.
- **Be cheerful and enthusiastic.** Now this is obviously not possible if you are sick, but the negative, whining person will drive away his or her cast of thousands.
- **Live in the present.** This means don't look too far down the road. We're not encouraged to be foolhardy and not prepare for the future, but if we look too far into the future, we miss the magic of the day.
- **Be tidy.** This might sound like a funny recommendation, but if we spend most of our life looking for things, obviously we've wasted lots of opportunity.
- **Within reason, try to be peaceful. Mend fences.** To be angry and

hostile and to lash out at friends and colleagues or at the system wastes lots of energy and is incredibly negative and counterproductive.

- **Be resourceful.** Figure out a way to make things happen.
- **Reach out to others.** No person can go it alone.
- **Delegate.** A comment was made about a prominent Jesuit theologian, Father John Powell. He became drained physically and spiritually exhausted and was unable to function. Why? He viewed himself as Atlas trying to hold up the world. We need to delegate. We need help, and this is especially true if you are ill.

Mindful retreats are my alternative medicine. My personal stress relief. You don't have to go somewhere to create your own mindful retreat. A few moments of meditation—a long soak in the bathtub, a brisk walk—capture the healing power of solitude and contemplation. I recommend it every day.

Music for the Body . . . Music for the Soul

I think music in itself is healing. It's an explosive expression of humanity. It's something we are all touched by.

—Billy Joel

Close your eyes and hum the theme from the movie *Jaws.* Is your heart beating faster? Do you feel fearful? Surely you pictured sharks in your mind's eye. You may not even be aware of the effect, but music can create a conditioned response. Interestingly, nuns in a convent who never saw the movie *Jaws* can listen to the same music and not picture sharks.

Imagine, now, the power of music to heal.

The principle behind behavior change with music builds on the work of seventeenth-century Dutch physicist Christian Huygens, who discovered that clocks placed next to each other would tick in synchrony. This natural rhythm or entrainment in which two bodies move together becomes apparent when the beat of music prompts you to physically slow your heart rate, release muscle tension, and deepen your breath, thus producing relaxation.

Certain music—like a meditation mantra—can calm you and help you unwind. And you can train yourself to consciously relax. Your heart rate will slow as it entrains with the rhythm of the music. Practice makes perfect, so every time you hear music that calms you (and it's different music for everyone), you can automatically trigger your relaxation response. If you are hospitalized, think about taking your Walkman or MP3 player or, if appropriate, a small bedside CD player and your favorite calming music. This may have some impact on your body's immune system and may help bring linkage and peace back to the mind–body connection.

This emerging discipline of music therapy is becoming more mainstream. Some of the more popular uses of this technique are in the hospice setting. Hospices are places where individuals may go with serious medical illnesses—many have hospice care in their own homes. The lifespan of people in hospice settings usually is expected to be less than twenty-four weeks. Music has become an integral therapy to calm the mind and calm the soul during these dark hours.

Now let's participate in the music itself. Certainly singing is one form of vocal music therapy, but a centuries-old technique called chanting is being practiced to generate mental and physical health benefits. Chanting is akin to singing, only you repeat the "song" over and over, either out loud or silently, alone or in a group.

Chanting helps you withdraw your mental focus from worldly matters. Chanting captures sound as vibration. Vibration creates power. For example, as high notes in song have been known to shatter crystal, chanting helps evoke the relaxation response, which is essential to meditation. Secondary benefits of chanting include regulating breathing, slowing the heart rate, evoking deeper concentration, and releasing helpful brain chemicals to elevate mood and energy levels.

Even without the meditation component of chanting, you can just chant in the shower or even in the car, as a way to insulate yourself from road rage during the daily commute. Experiment with special CDs recorded with chanting in various Eastern languages and using instruments such as the sitar. Practitioners say the more you do it, the better you'll feel.

It would be a leap of faith to state that music therapy will make serious diseases go away, but it certainly enhances quality of life and creates a sense of well-being.

There's Something About a Wagging Tail

"I need to get home to see Max," my patient told me. I thought he was talking about his son, Max, or Maxine, his wife. But it turns out he was talking about his dog, Max. That was his drive to overcome tragic illness and get out of the hospital.

If you were stranded on a deserted island, would you want the company of your pet or another human? More than half of people surveyed by the American Animal Hospital Association chose their pets. Think about it. Who's the first one at the front door when you come home?

We can no longer ignore the medical significance of the *bond* people have with their pets. Our pets create a balance between our minds and our bodies in the truest sense of mind–body medicine.

I suggest pets to some cancer patients to help them cope with the rigors of their disease. In fact, I consider getting a pet to be one of the easiest and most rewarding ways of living a longer, healthier life.

What is it about these creatures? The wagging tail, a soft purr or rub against your leg, the tranquility of swimming fish. This is unconditional love and utter devotion—and this is the only time money can buy it. Research continues to tell us that pets, in turn, keep their owners happy, healthy and active. My good friend Dr. Marty Becker, the engaging resident veterinarian on *Good Morning America,* has documented the healing power of the animal–human bond in his book, *The Healing Power of Pets.*

Marty and I have presented to audiences on the "pet prescription." Our unlikely tag team duo of cancer doctor and veterinarian is really not so incongruous. Both disciplines—medicine and veterinary medicine—can be part of the healing team.

Dog and cat people will understand why the pet prescription works in amazing ways. The medical research literature bears this out, so let me highlight what we know:

- When you stroke your pet, within minutes your brain releases a spa treatment of brain chemicals that makes you feel good—and your pet receives similar benefits too. "Heavy petting" creates a sensory reaction similar to what takes place when a mother nurses her baby. This type of therapeutic touch really works.
- Petting pets lowers blood pressure; perhaps that's why pet owners take less medication for high blood pressure and high cholesterol. This puts

pet owners at a reduced risk for heart disease. Even among people who suffered heart attacks, pet owners had a four times better chance of surviving one year than did those who did not have pets. For people with arthritic hands, massage your pet and you both feel better.

- People with AIDS who have pets are less likely to suffer from depression than others with AIDS who don't own pets.

- Some people's pets can alert them to low blood sugar if they have diabetes or can sense a heart attack or asthma attack coming on. These are rare animals who perform such life-saving activities. Don't trust your feline or poodle with this task, however.

- If you will recall the relaxation response discussed earlier, you can achieve that state of calm with pets as well. Especially if you have chronic pain, a pet can take your focus off your pain and elevate your mood. The physical contact with pets can block transmission of pain and shut down your pain centers. High-tech imaging has actually shown reduced blood flow in pain areas when the "pet prescription" is taken as directed.

- Pets keep you moving. Sometimes your best exercise partner is your dog. There's nothing like that Yorkie "look" or a nudge from a Labrador retriever's nose to get you off the couch and onto the sidewalk. Pet ownership, especially of dogs, gets you outside and into more social interactions. And you will recall the social connectedness theme I have been advocating. Walk your canine and meet your neighbors.

- Like a K-9-1-1, pets can buffer your reaction to acute stress, as well as diminish perceptions of stress. A few minutes alone with your cat or dog might do more to help your stress than talking about your troubles with a best (human) friend or spouse.

- Therapy animals, mostly dogs, are commonplace in hospitals and nursing homes. Why? Because they bring something we doctors can't find in pills. Medical-care centers are bringing in animal-assisted therapy teams—usually certified dogs and their well-trained humans—to go from room to room, bed to bed with their own gentle brand of just "being there" for patients.

- Pets bring measurable joy to people in long-term care facilities, too. Animal-assisted therapy effectively reduced the loneliness of residents who wished to receive the therapy. Many nursing-home residents have had a strong life history of relationships with pets as an intimate part of their support system. Perhaps that's why nurses have observed residents with Alzheimer's disease who had not spoken to daughters or sons or grandchildren talking animatedly with therapy golden retrievers. If given the choice (and many elderly cannot have pets where they live, which should be a defining factor when you seek a care facility for your loved ones), they would choose to continue that pet bond.

- Older people with pets do much better in warding off depression. They're better able to withstand social isolation. Having a pet helps them be more active. Lest you think that's because they take dogs for walks, cat owners showed an equally higher rate of life-enhancing activity. And I haven't seen many cats on walks lately.

- On the other end of the age spectrum, children undergoing dental or medical procedures will feel less pain when a dog is present—and not just at their side. Kids said procedures were less painful even when the dog was curled up in the corner of the exam room.

- It's not just a dog-and-cat world. People with physical, psychological, cognitive, social and behavioral problems such as cerebral palsy, developmental disabilities and depression, even chronic abuse and eating disorders, are learning the healing power of riding horses. (This is known as *hippotherapy* and has nothing to do with hippopotamuses.)

I've known many people whose health went rapidly downhill after their pet died. Marty tells me veterinarians have observed this same pattern. Often, a beloved pet might be the most significant factor in motivating a seriously ill person to stay alive.

For my patients, I make a note in their medical record of their pets' names. And when the patient returns to see me, I ask, "How's Reggie?" or "How's Boots?" I find that this really eases some patients' anxiety about coming back for treatment.

Pets have a positive influence on our health because we all need something to live for and something to focus on besides ourselves. Self-absorption is terrible for your health. Pets accept us, no matter what. This unconditional love is even better, say some research studies, than admiration of friends.

I think part of the reason we connect so strongly with animals in general, not just pets, may be their emotional depth. Elephants mourn, even cry. Non–pet owners are, by now, shaking their heads. But who can question the unselfish love a pet has for you? Pets depend on us. Family may not. And we all know it feels good to be needed.

Let me share with you a powerful story about the depth of the animal-human bond. Several years ago, I received a phone call from a close family member who is one of the most accomplished anesthesiologists at a major medical center. His specialty is cardiovascular anesthesia. He is responsible for the life-and-death decisions of patients receiving heart transplants. This is emotionally draining and physically demanding work. Some of these cases take eighteen to twenty hours.

When he called me, he was obviously shaken. I could hear his distress. He was inconsolable and the sobs were palpable through the phone. My initial thought was that a family member had died or there was some catastrophe at work. Not so. His beloved golden retriever, Sadie, had to be put to sleep. Sadie was a part of the household like children and parents. Sadie began losing weight and was taken to the veterinarian. The veterinarian suspected some minor liver ailment and advised an exploratory procedure. With the beloved animal sedated, the veterinarian was horrified to note that much of the abdominal cavity and the liver had been replaced by a highly virulent malignant tumor. All agreed that the best thing was to give Sadie the easy way out and euthanize her.

This was one of the most painful decisions of his life. It was especially painful because there was no one at work he could share this with. A man who held others' lives in his own hands every day was completely torn apart over his family dog.

This was my experience also with Molly, and perhaps you have had these defining moments as well. Molly was our beloved Lhasa Apso. A ten-pound creature who brought joy to each of our hearts. Then the ultimate irony struck. Molly developed malignant melanoma on the floor of the tongue with extensive involvement of the lungs, liver and brain. I will never forget the day that we brought her to the vet for her final trip. Her sad brown eyes looked up at us and basically said, "It is okay. You did your best. You gave me your best shot, and I now know what needs to be done."

We agonized over this decision for weeks. Her labored breathing, her obvious pain and her physical deterioration were clear signs that the end was in sight. Animals become part of our souls, and animals can take a piece of our soul, but that is simply the way life is. Animals can soothe our souls as well.

And now enter Brinkley.

A week or so before Christmas four years ago, my wife, Peggy, and I were called to see a little puppy at the animal shelter and to consider adopting him. It was a frigid December day with waist-deep snow. We trudged up the walk, and our lives were changed forever.

He was called Chance by the people at the shelter because that indeed was what his life was all about—another chance. One of a litter of golden retrievers, some accident had befallen him. His rear right leg was so badly injured, it had been amputated.

These big brown eyes—eyes of forgiveness, eyes of peace, eyes of compassion—looked up at us. Bingo, out came the checkbook and things have never been quite the same.

This little creature for whom life was very unfair offers unconditional love, unconditional acceptance and unconditional forgiveness. He has become somewhat of a TV star, having appeared on a local television station, and has become one of the stars of the Mayo Clinic Web site because his picture that accompanies our story on the healing power of puppy love has been amazingly popular.

Now where did the name Brinkley come from? For some reason the name Chance did not fit this little character, but if you've seen Meg Ryan in the charming movie *You've Got Mail*, we were struck by the final scene in which there is a beautiful golden retriever named Brinkley. It seemed so fitting for our star.

The take-home message: While we may have saved Brinkley's life, he really has saved ours. He gives us some of the best medicine money can buy. Our other family members include Jessie, a beautiful, fun-loving (and probably way too energetic) golden retriever, and Reggie, an orange tabby we adopted as a stray. I must say, Reggie is the smartest cat in the universe.

Not a Laughing Matter—Oh, but It Is

Can you find a healing punch at your neighborhood Blockbuster Video store? I think so.

Norman Cousins, longtime editor of the *Saturday Review* and faculty member at a medical school in California, wrote a fascinating book called *Anatomy of an Illness as Perceived by the Patient: Reflections on Healing and Regeneration*. Cousins was diagnosed with a severe type of arthritis involving his spine called ankylosing spondylitis. My sense is that Cousins was given a fairly grim prognosis. He realized in his own life the tremendous value of laughter in putting a more positive spin on a desperate situation.

He spent many hours watching movies with the Three Stooges and roared with the enthusiasm of an adolescent at some of the antics of Larry, Curly and Moe. Cousins indicates that his recovery was related, at least in part, to his ability to simply let go of the situation and let it unfold.

If you're looking forward to a favorite comedy on TV, just checking the TV listings may trigger healthy mood changes, reduce your stress hormone levels and boost your immune system's defenses.

A study presented at the Society for Neuroscience is the first to show that even anticipation of a mirthful event may be good for you. Lee Berk, assistant professor of family medicine, and his colleagues at the Susan Samueli Center for Complementary and Alternative Medicine at the University of California-Irvine, found that anticipating a laugh-inducing event reduced levels of tension, anger, depression, fatigue and confusion up to two days *before* the actual event.

Now why should humor be such a powerful tool? It is very clear that certain molecules or brain chemicals (endorphins), secreted from deep within the brain, trigger the placebo effect. These types of molecules achieve a high blood level during times of stress, such as running a marathon (the "runner's high") or when involved in an automobile accident. These hormones provide a feeling of wellness and euphoria and may have something to do with augmenting the immune system.

Should a comedian be part of the medical team? Obviously, that would not be appropriate. However, emerging studies from social science and psychology tell us a sense of lightheartedness not only acknowledges the futility of life but also underscores the humanity of the caregiver. Humor also acknowledges that in a very real sense we are all patients. We are simply at different points along the journey.

Patch Adams is a fascinating West Virginia physician who recognizes the incredible healing power of humor. Patch embraces the relative futility of what medicine can offer some patients. Sure, there have been great advances in technology and hardly a day goes by when some so-called breakthrough is not heralded in the media. However, a hunger in the soul of every patient is a bond or a connectedness with the physician. The physician who recognizes the humanity of the patient and of himself or herself has a unique gift to bring to the bedside.

Humor happens when you least expect it—even to me. On a bitterly cold January morning, I walked into an examining room. I reviewed the patient's history. It was clear that we were dealing with a desperate problem. The patient had a history of lung cancer, and the records from home indicated he was having some difficulties with weakness. After examining the man, it was obvious that the left side of his body was paralyzed. His arm flailed at his side. His left leg could not support any weight. He used a crutch under his right armpit to walk.

Together we looked at the MRI scan of his brain. It indicated a baseball-sized tumor. I explained that the tumor could not be surgically removed. We discussed some options, and it was most appropriate that we admit him to the hospital.

And now, the rest of the story.

The patient said to me, "Doc, what should I do with my dog and my truck?" I was dumbfounded. The patient told me that he had driven his truck with his dog riding shotgun for hundreds of miles, through the murderous freeways of Chicago, with a complete paralysis of the left side of his body!

He told me that the most difficult part of the journey was trying to aim his truck through the tollbooth. On his first attempt, he knocked out the left headlight. He later learned, through four more tollbooths, that if he got in the far right-hand lane, he could navigate through that maze. Unfortunately, his dog could not drive. The next challenge was to somehow stop the truck, put it in park, and, with his right hand, reach across his body to drop two quarters in the toll bucket. The human spirit should never be denied. We laughed so hard, we cried at the retelling of this story.

As the doctor and the patient and family become more comfortable and get to know each other, a bizarre and wonderful bond forms. For me, this is quite unlike the attachment in any other medical specialty because of the emotional impact of the type of medicine I specialize in. There are incredibly rich moments of lightheartedness that patients share with us during these tender times. All of a sudden, the Palm Pilot, the day planner, the elaborate time-management schemes fade by the wayside. Patients focus on each day as it arises and are able to see some of the absurdity in life.

A middle-aged farmer was dying from an advanced cancer. Prior to his illness he had been negotiating with a roofing contractor to replace the shingles on his farm home. The contractor he had finally selected offered him a fifty-year guarantee that not one shingle would ever need to be replaced. With a wry sense of humor, this patient finished the story, "Heck, Doc, I don't even have fifty days left let alone fifty years, but I got a good deal on the shingles."

My Thoughts . . .

We are all patients. We are simply at different points on the journey. We physicians can certainly understand the need of patients to seek out alternative practitioners. But I urge you to be realistic in your search for health, peace and serenity.

12

Attitude Matters: The Psychology of Survival and Longevity

*We cannot live only for ourselves. A thousand fibers
connect us with our fellow men; and among those fibers,
as sympathetic threads, our actions run as courses,
and they come back to us as effects.*

—Herman Melville

Bottom Line: You Can Survive Any Diagnosis

Almost every day in the clinic, I see patients who do not conform to what is described in medical textbooks. What I am trying to say is that these people had dreadful prognoses based upon a pathology report, a CT scan, or what we observed in the operating room, yet they have continued to do amazingly well.

We sample blood and look for patterns in their immunology. We perform a variety of tests on their hormones. But there does not seem to be a consistent theme from what we can see in the laboratory studies. Of course not. The answer to their success lies elsewhere. Each of these patients does seem to have several traits in common.

When I reviewed much of the world's medical literature on the subject of survival, three themes seemed to emerge with long-term survivors:

- **A sense of religion.** By this, I mean individuals participating in the set of rules and regulations for certain belief systems, faith-based, but not necessarily.
- **A sense of spirituality.** Many definitions exist for this term, but the one that seems to work for many of us is the questioning of the ultimate purpose of life: Why are we here? What is this all about? It is an attempt to find meaning, purpose and cohesion in a sea of chaos and confusion.
- **A sense of connectedness.** You know them. They are your parents, neighbors, coworkers and, I hope, you. These people typically have long-term meaningful adult relationships with spouses or partners, or are members of a community that gives them support and encouragement during times of crisis. The isolated individual, the disenfranchised "grumpy old man," generally does not do well when faced with adversity.

What Can We Learn from the Long-Term Survivor?

While having the privilege of being the attending physician on the Oncology Service at one of our hospitals, I have had a number of experiences that have brought home some solid, time-honored truths.

Let me set the scene. The oncology ward consists of about twenty-five to thirty patients, most of whom have far-advanced malignant disease. Some of them were admitted to the hospital for the evaluation and management of complications related to their cancer treatments, which included nausea, vomiting, pain and related miseries.

Fortunately, with aggressive management many of these symptoms can be controlled so the patients can spend the remaining time in relative comfort and dignity.

As I make rounds in the hospital and visit with these patients and their families, several observations are noteworthy:

- On the nightstand next to the patient's hospital bed, I do not see stock portfolios, certificates of achievement or an acknowledgment of having been a good and faithful corporate soldier. What I do see are snapshots of children, grandchildren and pets, wedding pictures, and religious mementos such as Bibles, rosaries and related accessories.
- The discussions I have with these patients never focus on accomplishments, achievements and the size of one's wealth. Discussions almost always focus on missed opportunities, remorse and regrets, and "what I would have done if I had more time."
- What I hear from many patients and their families is the ache in their souls concerning what might have been, what could have been and how they should spend their remaining time.
- We each need programs, projects and proposals to get us out of bed on a Monday morning. When faced with life-ending illness, the paycheck becomes irrelevant. We need to contribute, we need to feel part of a greater good, and finally we need to remember that each of us has the gifts and skills to make the world a little kinder, a little softer, a little better than it is right now.

Who are these patients—these heroes of everyday life? We see them everywhere. These are the anonymous faces of simple citizens who somehow continue to thrive in the face of life's unfairness, who continue to somehow dodge the bullets fired from the barrels of poverty, alcohol, abusive relationships and just plain bad luck.

- The young single mom working the swing shift in a factory
- The midlife homemaker suffering in silence from the anguish of divorce and a bitter custody battle
- The seasoned executive banished by an MBA younger than his son to a professional gulag where the only exits are a gold watch (actually gold-plated), a heart attack or a forced early retirement

Yet, somehow, people like these continue to suit up every day, tough it out, and have productive and meaningful lives. Now add a serious, life-threatening illness or injury to someone's life. Does everything stop? Or do we march on, suit up and give it our best shot?

What can we learn from the long-term survivor of a dread disease or serious injury or accident?

A lot. The hacking cough that doesn't quite go away; that vague indigestion accompanied by weight loss; a heart attack; a stroke; the brain injury that causes coma; the painless lump—each can be the start of a journey of terror and fear. Every patient's nightmare: "I'm sorry to tell you that you have cancer." "Your father has suffered a stroke; he will have a long road to rehabilitation and may never regain his ability to talk." "You have multiple sclerosis." "Your son has had a serious car accident and injured his brain." At one time, this clearly signaled the end of the road for many patients.

But not today.

Patients are living longer than ever before with diseases and injuries that would have brought premature death to their parents or grandparents just a few decades ago. The proportion of long-term cures and medical marvels continues to increase, and for the patient who cannot be cured, there have been major advances in managing the symptoms and complications of the disease and also the treatment.

> *The longer I live, the more I realize the impact of attitude on life. Attitude . . . is more important than facts, it is more important than the past, than education, than money, than circumstances, than failures, . . . [attitude] will make or break a company . . . a church . . . a home. The remarkable thing is we have a choice every day regarding the attitude we will embrace for that day. We cannot change our past. . . . The only thing we can do is play on the one string we have, and that is our attitude. I am convinced that life is 10 percent what happens to me and 90 percent how I react to it. . . . We are in charge of our attitudes.*
>
> —Charles Swindoll

A tale of two patients

The date: December 12. The year: 1999. The place: Room 4162 on the cancer unit. Two patients in adjoining beds have identical diagnoses. Each has advanced cancer of the pancreas, which had spread into the liver. Cancer of the pancreas is one of the most virulent and aggressive cancers. The average survival is limited to a few short months in those circumstances.

Each patient was told about the need for recovery following surgery, and a follow-up appointment was made for one month after dismissal from the hospital. One patient returned looking miraculously well, even though the cancer had slightly progressed. On the other hand, the other patient had markedly deteriorated with profound weakness, weight loss and an unraveling quality of life. What was the difference in the course of these two patients? This is the sort of question that makes medicine fascinating.

I asked the obviously well patient what he did to try to keep this monster under control. Here was his game plan:

- He left the hospital with the following questions and challenge to his health-care providers: "What can I do as a patient? What can my family do to give me the best odds of squeezing out a few extra months from this cancer? I want to participate. I want to be in charge. I do not simply want to sit back and take advice."
- With this attitude, the patient sought the guidance of a physical therapist concerning an appropriate and aggressive program of stretching, reasonable exercise and walking. He sought the input of a registered dietitian on some dos and don'ts and general guidelines about nutrition.
- He made a list of what was really important for him now that the clock was ticking. He jettisoned some community committee responsibilities. He gracefully exited from some commitments at work. He focused only on the one or two functions that were important to him, such as the Rotary Club and his weekly poker group.
- He informed himself about the reasonable anticipated natural history of his illness, and he clearly understood the limitations and possible side effects of treatment.

Now what about the patient who was struggling for survival? What did he do? This patient did none of the above. He had a stoic, "Western frontier" mentality and thought he could go it alone, much like the Lone Ranger. He became isolated from his family and friends. He did not have a list of priorities. He simply accepted what he heard about his diagnosis.

We need to be realistic. It is not possible to wish away advanced disease. Nor is it reasonable to buy a lottery ticket instead of planning for retirement. But you can place your energy and emphasis on the psychological, spiritual and social dimension of life so that you can gently shift the odds in your favor to squeeze out a few more quality weeks or months from a serious illness.

Keys to the kingdom

When embroiled in the dark days of World War II, Winston Churchill rallied his countrymen and women: "Never give in, never give in, never, never, never, never . . ."

With those words, he galvanized the spirit and the energies of the British people and helped sustain them in their valiant battle against Nazi Germany. This sort of philosophy has been used by many a coach as a team dismally fell behind at halftime. Sometimes it worked, but most of the time, I suspect, these sorts of speeches have little impact in an athletic contest. Now, let's turn our focus to an interesting medical situation.

At the present time in the war against cancer, it is appropriate and fashionable to offer groups of patients a certain treatment, let's say immunotherapy, to determine the benefit of the treatment among those individuals. In general, we hope to see benefit in approximately 20 percent of patients. When that occurs, there is encouragement to open that treatment to far greater numbers of patients. This is called a clinical trial. The assessment of an anticancer treatment among hundreds of patients gives us a good "feel" for the ultimate value of that treatment. However, the flip side of that coin sometimes is not appreciated. Not every patient will be helped. These brave souls go into clinical trials with great expectations and hopes.

It is my recollection that almost every great advance in medicine or surgery was generated by the observation of one physician dealing with one patient. The curiosity of that individual fueled additional studies and helped pave the way for some important advances. Penicillin is a case in point. Sir Alexander Fleming happened to drop some moldy bread into a dish of bacteria. Lo and behold, the bacteria were killed. Penicillin was discovered. These sorts of observations make history. Now let me tell you about an interesting fellow.

The patient was a gentleman in his mid-forties who went for a routine examination. He was feeling generally well. To the dismay of his examining physician, there was a mass in the rectal area. A biopsy confirmed it as malignant melanoma. The patient underwent a CT scan of the abdomen. There were extensive tumors in the liver and in the chain of lymph nodes surrounding the aorta. Under most circumstances, this would be viewed as a hopeless, dismal problem. The patient and his enormously supportive wife decided to receive investigational chemotherapy in a clinical trial. It had no benefit. He was not in the small group of patients to receive benefit from the drug being tested.

As the disease relentlessly progressed, the patient was willing to proceed with "off-the-shelf" chemotherapy, which traditionally had virtually no chance of helping. The treatment was offered during a summer, and the patient was not expected to survive. Well, that was our expectation.

Much to our amazement, shortly after the Vikings victory in the NFL playoffs, the patient called for an appointment! We were amazed and gratified that he was still with us. The patient and his wife suggested additional scans, and we discovered that the cancer was in remission. It was still present but had not spread. His physical examination also confirmed that there was very little obvious evidence of cancer.

Now, what do we make of this observation? Is it a miracle? Is it simply a roll of the dice? Does it have something to do with the alignment of the planets? Obviously, any or all or none of these explanations may be adequate, but this gentleman does have some of the characteristics of long-term cancer survivors—a sense of connectedness with his devoted wife and a reason for living.

So far, we do not have a brain-wave test for survival. Nor can we perform an MRI of the head or devise a psychiatric profile that can predict "up front" which people will do well. But I do think that, when faced with a serious problem, the words of Winston Churchill ("Never give up") are very reasonable to consider. We must embrace the harsh reality that these types of exceptional stories are most unusual, but at some point in history, these patients may provide the keys to the kingdom to help us really understand why some people do better than others.

A recent review published in the *British Medical Journal* analyzed twenty-six studies on the effective psychological coping styles and survival from cancer or its reoccurrence. The authors found little convincing evidence that attitude and disposition play a role in surviving malignant disease.

Contrary to this review, it has been my clinical experience and that of many colleagues that **we cannot discount or cast aside the relationship between the mind and the body.** I cannot dismiss my own review of the research on long-term cancer survivors (and for that matter, it could be survivors of any other life-threatening illness) plus research showing that pessimists have a 19 percent shorter life span than optimists.

So what does this all mean? It means that we in traditional medicine do not have all the answers, and it also means that a portfolio of coping skills including the sense of spirituality and the sense of community and connectedness must be part of a comprehensive disease treatment program to give patients the best chance of beating the odds.

Traditionally, medicine and religion were bonded to each other. During the fifth century, most physicians were members of the clergy. By the Middle Ages, the church had the ultimate authority over medical practices and awarded "licenses" to practice medicine.

One of the driving forces of this relationship was the obvious lack of understanding of physiology and biology. By the 1800s, a mechanical-biomedical model emerged as a result of advances in pathophysiology. This led to a period of so-called enlightenment in which medical illness did not reflect punishment or moral inadequacy. Attempts were made to explain virtually all human sickness on the basis of biochemical or pathophysiologic mechanism. In other words, individuals who contracted tuberculosis died of that infection. Individuals who had a heart attack and had blocked coronary arteries died from their illness. However, we now understand that not all patients with tuberculosis die and not all patients with heart attacks die, so there must be some other emotional and psychological factors to help explain this finding.

This old notion of illness of the body did not consider the profound importance of emotional, spiritual and psychosocial factors affecting human illness. The medical community now recognizes that the vast majority of patients have disorders that are clearly related to emotional issues rather than to physical disease.

This fundamental concept was articulated in 1931 by Dr. William J. Mayo, who wrote: "The failure [of the medical profession] lies in an [in]ability to appreciate and deal intelligently with the emotional instabilities of those physically ill . . . which lead to miseries as grievous as though they were dependent on tangible physical causes."

Thus we ask the question: What is the influence of emotional and spiritual elements on disease?

Mind–Body–Spirit Connection

We oncologists have at our command the most spectacular advances in immunology, imaging and therapy for cancer. Yet we feel a nagging uneasiness that something is missing in our healing quiver. A flood of books called our attention to the mind–body–spirit connection and discussed how the gravely ill patient can harness this concept to enhance quality of life and perhaps even survival.

During the mid-1980s, Bernie Siegel's book *Love, Medicine, and Miracles: Lessons Learned about Self-Healing from a Surgeon's Experience with Exceptional Patients* appeared in hospital rooms throughout the United States. This was an important work because it discussed patient involvement in dealing with cancer. He championed a heightened sense of responsibility. He encouraged patients to be active participants in treatment decisions. Patients were appropriately invited to challenge the medical institution itself and were advised not to be passive participants swept away by the armada of medical technology.

Eventually, this positive message became distorted. Some authors suggested that the "fighters"—patients who tenaciously engaged their doctors in alternative practices—and the "optimists" would somehow be granted a reprieve from their illness.

This misguided philosophy placed a dreadful burden on the shoulders of each patient. I saw this among my cancer patients, and I suspect it holds true for other specialists in their medical fields.

Simply, the faulty message was this: Because you are responsible for your health and wellness, and because attitude is important in your well-being, if your cancer progresses or if treatment is ineffective, this clearly means you are not trying hard enough. Somehow, it's your fault if the cancer progresses. **This is simply not true.**

A more recent book, Larry Dossey's *Meaning & Medicine: Lessons from a Doctor's Tales of Breakthrough and Healing* underscores the importance of thoughts, emotions, and meaning in health and illness, especially about cancer. Dr. Dossey's message here is that what a patient thinks has an important effect on well-being. In other words, a cause and effect. And chapters with titles such as The Power of Belief, Healing at a Distance, and The Invisible Power Within posed interesting medical questions that cannot be answered by our current methods of scientific inquiry.

In the pages of Dr. Dossey's book and others, patients offer personal testimonials, and medical practitioners tell about their observations among patients—somehow implying that attitude and disposition can bring about physical cures and miracles. Again, the burden of responsibility rests squarely with the patients, and I see that as a dangerous idea.

We can thank these books for one thing. They created a sensitivity and awareness about the fact that patients have a responsibility to be active partners with their caregivers. But by placing the responsibility for wellness on the patients and ignoring the fact that cancer and other diseases are also a biological process—and patients don't have control over that—these books are creating a dark downside.

Where's the Scientific Proof?

More recently, authors of similar books are relying less on stories from single patients and are performing credible research to document the value of the mind–body–spirit connection objectively. In fact, Caryle Hirshberg, the author of *Remarkable Recovery: What Extraordinary Healings Tell Us About Getting Well and Staying Well,* posed these questions:

- When faced with a life-altering disease, can you do anything to modify the natural history of that event?
- Can you change any behaviors to enhance quality and possibly length of life?

The authors talked to long-term survivors to pinpoint the characteristics of these remarkable people and discovered some common threads:

- Long-term survivors seemed to reach a spiritual dimension through prayer or meditation.
- Long-term survivors held an innate belief that somehow the situation would be all right.
- Long-term survivors were connected either to a spouse or life partner or to a community. In fact, some had long-term marriages lasting more than thirty years.

Now, these characteristics are not a blueprint or a guarantee for survival, but they suggest that long-term survivors are not simply "lucky people" either. It also says to me that some factors influencing the outcome of cancer or other life-threatening illness can be modified.

So what does this mean? It means that some patients with dreadful conditions do amazingly well. We do not yet have the specific probes of their personalities, but we do know that social isolation is a significant factor in mortality, and study after study shows that individuals with a sense of community and connectedness do better than individuals who are marginalized, disenfranchised and isolated.

We must remember that although biology is destiny, we can tinker with some things in life to enhance the quality of life.

Connectedness:
The Importance of Social Support

Cherish your human connections: your relationships with friends and family.

—Barbara Bush

Let's look harder at what it means to have connectedness in life. David Spiegel, M.D., Stanford psychiatrist and author of *Living Beyond Limits: New Hope and Help for Facing Life-Threatening Illness,* divided a group of women with far-advanced breast cancer into two sections: Half met weekly and participated in a support group. The other half were not in a support group. The findings were striking.

The women who had the weekly support did far better, in terms of survival, than the individuals who were by themselves. This was an intriguing study but was viewed with some skepticism. There were some statistical flaws in the trial well acknowledged by Dr. Spiegel, and until a confirmatory study is published, the jury is still out on the value of support groups in prolonging survival from cancer. But there is no question that under proper circumstances these support groups empower patients and enhance quality of life.

I commonly ask some of these remarkable patients the reason for their striking survival in the face of impossible odds. The responses of these patients are predictable. First, there is a laugh of embarrassment and awkwardness. Second, patients typically use a joke or sarcasm: "Oh, I don't know. I guess I am too mean and too nasty to leave this Earth."

But then they share with me the rest of the story. In almost every circumstance, it is a relationship, a person or a pet that motivates the patient to push on and trudge forward in face of impossible odds. A newly born grandchild, a horse that is now part of their stable or a renewed relationship with a long-lost sibling are the kinds of stories that we hear over and over again. Interestingly, none of these patients has been driven by the need to increase his or her portfolio, magnify their 401(k) plan or enhance their net worth. Things, trinkets are irrelevant. Relationships and connectedness were common threads in the lives of each of these individuals.

Now is this a scientific study? Of course not, but we need to recognize that almost every advance in medicine has been made by the observation of a curious clinician visiting with a remarkable patient and questioning, wondering, and then looking for truth.

I'm not surprised by the power of connectedness. Friends may be able to persuade patients with illness to eat right, exercise regularly and listen to their doctors' advice. And while others have championed the fighter and the optimist as being best-suited to deal with cancer, it may be that these people simply have a social support system to buffer them against stress and to help them cope with their medical care. Their attitudes may have nothing to do with their illness and everything to do with seeking friends to support them during difficult times.

The Debate Continues

The greatest healing therapy is friendship and love.
—Hubert H. Humphrey

Social scientists have long recognized that we have survived as a species because of our ability to band together in small clans and colonies to fight enemies, to keep ourselves warm and dry, and to feed our young. Studies of entire populations consistently make some rather interesting observations:

- People who lack social relationships are at higher risk of death.
- Socially isolated people have an increased risk of dying.
- Being married is a plus for your health. Losing a spouse through death is not good for your health, especially for men.

The specific reasons why social relationships make a difference in whether you have good health or die early are unclear. But let's speculate.

Social relationships probably influence health, either by promoting a sense of meaning and purpose in life, which enhances health, or by bringing about positive lifestyle habits in terms of sleep, nutrition and exercise.

Let me mention a few more scientific studies to make this point. One study looked at African American and white women with breast cancer. Race made no difference here. But the women who had few close personal ties or people they could turn to for emotional support had an increased death rate. These findings reinforced an earlier, similar study in which stress impaired the activity of natural defensive cells among patients with breast cancer.

So what should a newly diagnosed patient with a life-threatening illness do? If he is feeling socially isolated, should he run out and try to muster all the friends he can? Does she renew old friendships at the class reunion and hope some of them stick around to shepherd her through a period of treatment and recovery?

One of the classic models of support groups has been Alcoholics Anonymous. This has been a life-saving intervention for many men and women struggling with chemical dependency. This model has been expanded to virtually every ailment that affects humankind.

Is a support group right for you?

This is a highly individual decision. As a rule of thumb, people in the chemical-dependency world have suggested that it takes attendance at four to six meetings to get a sense and a feel for the program. You can quickly decide if the group "feels right" and is good for you. You must be mindful of comparing your case to another because each individual requires different management.

Return for a moment to the fascinating study by Dr. Spiegel and the support groups for women with breast cancer. There was a doubling of survival in the women who met every week for approximately one year compared with women who were not part of a support group. This advantage was highly statistically significant. But we need to look at the rest of the story.

In a scientific sense, the study was not strictly randomized. This means that a flip of a coin or a computer did not randomly assign women to one group or the other. Therefore, it is possible that the women who met every week were healthy enough, fit enough and had a social support system that encouraged them to join in the meeting. On the other hand, the women who did not meet on a regular basis were perhaps too ill or too fragile to do so. We also do not know about the support systems of the women who were not randomized to the group meeting each week. The verdict is still out on whether or not support systems increase length of life, but the success of these programs in most circumstances strongly suggests that the quality of life and the sense of community and connectedness cannot be ignored.

Now that I've told you what might work, let me flip the coin. Not all studies and researchers agree. In yet another study of breast cancer patients, the study participants were asked question after question about anxiety, worry, depression, social health, mental health, self-esteem and health beliefs. In this case, nothing predicted survival. Nothing. And the researchers concluded that the disease itself outweighed the influence of any psychosocial factors in determining survival.

Patients in another study were asked extensively about their faith, religion and attitude (the optimist versus the pessimist), and about the emotional stress they felt. Again, nothing seemed to predict survival—nothing except the biological progression of the life-threatening disease.

Separating Spirituality from Mind and Body

You have to accept whatever comes, and the only important thing is that you meet it with courage and the best you have to give.
—Eleanor Roosevelt

The element of spirituality, at least for oncologists, is slowly and subtly emerging. Slowly, because we cannot see it. Subtly, because we cannot measure it. But let me assure you, spirituality is the subject of many a professional meeting and more than a handful of scientific papers.

An often-cited study looked at the effects of intercessory prayer. I mentioned a similar study in the discussion about complementary medicine. This one is a little different. Patients who were admitted to a coronary-care unit were randomly assigned to an intervention or a control group. People who didn't know the patients, and who were not even at the bedside, prayed for the patients in the intervention group. For some of you, the outcome will be difficult to understand, and I suggest we view the results with caution. But the patients who were prayed for at a distance by strangers seemed to have better outcomes after their heart attacks.

This is an intriguing notion—a group of individuals in one location prays for an individual perhaps living in a different state or a different community. Some of these studies have demonstrated that the individuals who were prayed for did better than those who were not prayed for.

On the other hand, a major Mayo Clinic study addressing this situation did not convincingly show the value of intercessory prayer. However, the power of prayer can be a source of tremendous comfort for many people, and perhaps their thinking might go something like this. If an individual is ill and does know that people are praying for him or her, that individual obviously has a sense of community and connectedness. There is a sense that "at least somebody out there cares about me." And this sense of community and connectedness might be the driving factor behind why some patients who are prayed for might do better than those who are left to their own devices.

Now what happens to those of us who may not have families, who may be elderly, and who may not have a sense of community or connectedness? There are no quick fixes, there are no easy answers, but certainly, access to community resources—visiting nurses, Meals on Wheels and hospice programs, for example—should not be neglected. Many studies have shown that the mortality among widowers within a year of a wife having died is much higher than individuals who remain in committed long-term relationships not severed by death. I think this should tell us that by our nature we are communal beings. We were not destined to be isolated, and those who are not part of a community are at exceptionally high risk for significant adverse health consequences.

Every one of my colleagues and I have a group of patients who should have died years ago. We can't just say they are lucky. Clearly, connectedness and spirituality often are factors. But that is not the end of the story. Continued research may tell us more.

Of Hope and Guilt

If you can't change your fate, change your attitude.

—Amy Tan

Several years ago, Dr. Barri Cassileth published a study in *The New England Journal of Medicine*. She addressed the role of attitude and disposition among the terminally ill. The paper could show no benefit of attitude whatsoever, and this resonates with an even more recent study in the *British Medical Journal* and reported in the press with this headline: *Positive mental attitude does not affect cancer survival*.

How do we reconcile these findings with the general belief that attitude has something to do with illness?

An analogy might go something like this: If you are run over by a bus or a herd of buffalo, then it is highly unlikely that attitude and disposition have anything to do with survival because the assault on your body is completely overwhelming, and you are unable to respond. On the other hand, if you have an injury such as twisting your knee while skiing, or if you have the diagnosis of cancer and your psychological defenses are firmly rooted, then it seems logical that you may be able to marshal resources to better cope with the illness or injury. However, we need to recognize that we were genetically engineered to travel in packs and live in groups. The calf who becomes isolated from the herd has a very low probability of making it to adulthood.

Remarkable patients can make the point even better:

- A Midwestern farmer had a malignant melanoma removed from his lip and had multiple spots in his lungs. He was given a dismal prognosis at his local hospital. I gave him options and alternatives, and he shared with me what these options really gave him: hope. He explained that this gave him the possibility of a reprieve. At that point, everything became crystal-clear with vibrant colors. The sky was a vivid blue. The flowers were virtually iridescent, and everything had a Technicolor, almost three-dimensional look, feel and smell. He shared with me a sense of guilt that he was spared, whereas other good people in similar situations succumbed from their advanced cancers.

- Another middle-aged gentleman was diagnosed with an invasive, aggressive form of malignant melanoma—first spotted by his barber. The patient came to me in the middle 1980s and underwent appropriate surgery. Under the microscope this cancer had ominous characteristics and should have taken his life within a few months. That was fifteen years ago. The patient has done well financially and professionally but has a nagging angst that he was being spared for some greater good and some greater purpose, which is not yet clear to him.

- A prominent researcher from a well-known university is one of the foremost international academic superstars in a very narrow area of science. In the early 1980s, this researcher developed bone marrow metastasis from a malignant melanoma associated with skin lesions. The researcher received an experimental program of treatment. Nineteen of the twenty patients who participated in this trial died. She alone remains alive and well almost seventeen years later. Why? The patient was accustomed to and needed the challenge of getting through the rigors of an academic environment to survive. These characteristics served her well in dealing with her disease. This is the kind of individual who would wither if abandoned on a deserted island with no sense of purpose.

- A delightful young woman developed nasal congestion. Extensive evaluations showed an angry, aggressive, high-grade cancer arising from the base of her skull. The cancer could not be removed, and it had spread to the lungs. The patient is still alive almost twenty years later. Again, a sense of connectedness and purpose and a need to be present for her young children were clearly factors in her survival of a situation in which others died.

- In the mid-1980s, a factory worker from a rural area came to me with abdominal pain. He underwent an exploratory procedure in which one of our premiere abdominal surgeons detected a baseball-sized mass and multiple malignant satellites with the melanoma encasing the bowel. The patient underwent surgery to remove as much of the widespread cancer as possible, but it was clearly understood that a cancer was undoubtedly left behind. Again, the survival should have been no more than a few months. He likewise did well and continues to do well for fifteen-plus years. Queried as to why he did well, the patient indicated, "Somehow I just knew that I would beat this thing." Naive? No, I don't think so. More like a belief and a confidence that there was a higher power or cosmic force protecting him.

Each of these individuals provides thought-provoking insights into the resiliency of the human spirit. Psychologist Dr. Martin Seligman has extensively written about learned optimism. The optimists of life view setbacks and catastrophes as being transient, as being very specific—a bankruptcy, for example—and do not extrapolate the setbacks to all life's issues. He makes a valid point that I can speak to in these patients.

When someone receives an overwhelming diagnosis, the immune system, the soul and cognitive or higher functions simply cease to function. Some people never get over this "funk," and their depression is intertwined with an impairment of their immunity. They succumb to their illness. The optimists, somehow, have an inner spirit and inner drive to overcome adversity. This can be learned. This is not necessarily a genetically "done deal."

Now, how do we explain the phenomenon of the patient who is highly motivated, has a solid system of support and community, and has every reason to continue to live, yet he or she succumbs to the disease? What's the explanation then?

I don't think we know why this happens in some people, and this simply reflects our ignorance about the subtleties of the mind–body connection and the need for further research and studies in this area. Nevertheless, we cannot ignore the growing legion of patients who have survived far longer than anyone would have anticipated from their operative and pathology reports.

Now some tantalizing clues have been found from animal tumor experiments. When animals, whether they are rodents or primates or dogs, are given an electric shock in an experimental setting *and* the ability to control the shock to escape from the noxious environment, those animals do well. However, when the animals are exposed to relentless pressures, relentless stresses over which they have no control, the immune system clearly deteriorates. When these animals have tumors, their survival is drastically reduced.

This means that stress has something to do with the immune system and has something to do with survival. It is a small piece of the puzzle. As investigations continue, we may have better probes to precisely understand the mind–body connection.

THE FOUR BIG QUESTIONS

What gives your life enduring meaning?
What is the purpose of life?
What gets you out of bed on Monday morning?
What brings you joy?

How You Can Help Someone with a Serious Illness

John Donne said, "No man is an island." What he was really saying is that we are each part of the community. We are part of a family in a very general sense. In modern times, families may be blood relatives such as brothers and sisters and mothers and fathers. However, many of us are in a family or in a community of non–blood relatives. Now what does this mean for the patient?

From the time of antiquity, we survived by living in packs or groups. Lost creatures, separated from the pack, rarely survive alone. Likewise, from ancient scriptures, we are told that the individual who falls and has no one to carry him will perish.

High drama is played out in our hospitals every day. In most circumstances, patients have family members with them. In general, the support system can be a tremendous asset.

The family can be a remarkable ally and comfort to the patient, but families can also play a negative role. Let's look at some of the things that families can do to support and encourage patients during the journey of their lifetimes:

- **Be present.** This means simply showing up. But: "I don't know what to say." "I don't know how I can help." You don't have to do anything. The simple act of showing up and being present and acknowledging the person's illness can work wonders for the spirit and for the soul. Ask if the patient would like you to be present when the health-care team visits. Some people clutch their privacy like a child clutches a favorite teddy bear. Others wish to have another set of ears to hear what the nurses and doctors are saying. If you are asked to leave, don't make a scene but do so quietly. If you are asked to stay, explain later what you heard from the health-care team. Use simple language, don't embellish, and share with the patient your interpretations of what was said.
- **Understand that you are not the patient.** What you might wish for yourself during this time of turmoil might not be best for the patient. It is easy to be a hero when you are not in a foxhole and not on the firing line. The nauseated, pain-wracked patient with multiple sleepless nights is hardly in an ideal position to make a treatment decision, so be respectful of how that patient feels.

- **Know when it is time to show up, and know when it is time to leave.** Patients get tired. Patients are sick. Ask the patient about the best time for visits. Please understand that fighting disease or injury is an exhausting business and trying to maintain a stiff upper lip and happy façade for visitors takes lots of energy. Don't be discouraged and don't be offended if patients don't want to be involved in the usual chatter about the football season, the weather and the current race for mayor. These discussions become insignificant when faced with the eleventh hour of illness.
- **Ask the patient what you can bring him or her.** A favorite magazine. A favorite book or video can be far more important medicine than the kind that comes in bottles. Don't ever forget the power and the energy from a card, a thoughtful e-mail, the flowers or the baked lasagna. A box of cookies lines the stomach and warms the soul.
- **Be there for the long-term.** Make certain that the patient understands that you will be there whether the news is good or bad. As the journey unfolds, well-wishers quietly disappear. Sometimes, when the patient is most in need of support, the cast of thousands dwindles to a small number. Be among those who are counted when the going gets tough.

My Thoughts . . .

I have had the privilege of interacting with thousands of patients over my thirty-year career, and some are particularly memorable. Although all are courageous, some are particularly courageous.

You met Chris in the foreword of this book. I first met this young man in the early 1990s. He had positive lymph nodes being replaced by malignant melanoma under his armpit. The probability of survival then was zero. He returned to see me at three-month intervals, now every six months, and remains well today. When I visited with him recently, I entered the room and tears welled in my eyes as I saw him, his wife and his newborn baby flanked by his mother-in-law and mother. The sense of needing and purpose and of "being needed" were undoubtedly factors in his survival.

Twelve years ago, there were no proven therapies for Chris's situation, and the experimental treatments were not very promising. After thoughtful discussions with him and his family, we all agreed that proactive, aggressive surveillance with a careful history and physical exam and appropriate scans every several months would be reasonable. Today, he continues to see me. He's an established professional in his career. He has a lovely, supportive wife, a wonderful family and two beautiful sons. What is the lesson?

I do not have all the answers, but I can tell you that attitude, disposition and a supportive environment have something to do with surviving cancer or any life-threatening illness. We all recognize that some studies do not show the impact of attitude and disposition, but we cannot ignore these remarkable patients who defy the odds and somehow live meaningful, productive and creative lives in the face of a devastating prognosis. Chris and others defy the odds, rewrite the books, and provide hope and inspiration for us all.

Also at play here were early diagnoses, careful decision making about treatment, a savvy patient willing to make important lifestyle changes, a supportive family, a superb doctor–patient relationship—all key to navigating a changing medical system, to living a healthy life and to surviving any diagnosis—my message to you in this book. Thank you for reading. I now urge you to make meaningful lifestyle changes and be vigilant about your health . . . so you will not be my patient.

NEXT STEPS

Curious readers, you will want to pursue additional resources in your quest for health information. Let me give you some starting points. This list is certainly not comprehensive, as nothing in cyberspace can ever be.

Web Sites

The World Wide Web is a wonderful thing. Or it can be simply horrible. The Internet is changing the doctor–patient relationship. Use common sense and the guidelines from the National Center for Complementary and Alternative Medicine to judge the information you find online.

As always, any resource like this that publishes Web addresses becomes dated quickly. We apologize if any of these URLs have become broken links. As of publication, they were current.

Federal Government Sources

National Center for Complementary and Alternative Medicine (*www.nccam.nih.gov*)

Ten Things to Know About Evaluating Medical Resources on the Web (*www.nccam.nih.gov/health/webresources*)

Healthfinder (*www.healthfinder.gov*)—a key resource for finding the best federal government and nonprofit resources, links to hundreds of health-related organizations

U.S. Department of Health and Human Services (*www.health.gov*)—a portal to many government agencies and health initiatives, including the Surgeon General and the National Health Information Center

National Cancer Institute (*www.cancer.gov*)—extensive information on cancer research and clinical trials

PubMed (*www.ncbi.nlm.nih.gov/entrez/query.fcgi*)—the National Library of Medicine's ultimate search site for more than 12 million abstracts and citations in the scientific literature, dating back to the 1960s

Federal Citizen Information Center (*www.pueblo.gsa.gov*)—a one-stop consumer information center from the federal Government Services Administration; viewable and downloadable brochures and information on many topics, not just health

MEDLINEplus (*www.nlm.nih.gov/medlineplus*)—from the National Library of Medicine, information pages help you research your medical questions; extensive information on specific diseases and conditions; links to consumer health information, clearinghouses, dictionaries, lists of hospitals and physicians, health information in Spanish and other languages, and clinical trials

Food and Drug Administration (FDA) (*www.fda.gov*)—consumer information on prescription and over-the-counter drugs regulated by the federal government; use the MedWatch feature to report adverse drug reactions

National Women's Health Information Center, Office on Women's Health (*http://4woman.gov*)—from the Department of Health and Human Services, a gateway to federal and other women's health information sources

Centers for Disease Control and Prevention (CDC) (*www.cdc.gov*)—agency that promotes health and quality of life by preventing and controlling disease, injury and disability; resources on diseases, conditions, and other special topics such as travelers' health, immunizations and worldwide disease outbreaks

ClinicalTrials.gov (*http://clinicaltrials.gov*)—National Institutes of Health through the National Library of Medicine provides current information about clinical research trials actively recruiting patients for studies on all types of diseases

USDA Food and Nutrition Information Center (*www.nal.usda.gov/fnic*) —a gateway site to food safety, the Food Guide Pyramid, and dietary guidelines

Medical and Academic Centers

Mayo Clinic (*www.MayoClinic.com*)—my favorite place to start any medical search on any health subject; straightforward lifestyle and disease management centers, decision support tools; not surprising that this site appears on most top-ten lists

Aetna Intelihealth (*www.intelihealth.com*)—a supersite featuring consumer health information from Harvard Medical School

Harvard Center for Cancer Prevention (*www.yourcancerrisk. harvard.edu*)—Your Cancer Risk calculator estimates your risk

Memorial Sloan-Kettering Cancer Center (*www.mskcc.org*)—diagnosis and treatment information; also see the Information Resource: About Herbs, Botanicals and Other Products (*www.mskcc.org/aboutherbs*)

Oncolink, University of Pennsylvania Cancer Center (*www. oncolink.upenn.edu*)—a global resource for cancer information

University of Iowa's Virtual Hospital (*www.vh.org*)—a digital health sciences library created in 1992; for medical reference and health promotion

eMedicine.com (*www.eMedicine.com*)—access to the minds of medicine; peer-reviewed medical textbook–type information, updated instantly; written for medical professionals and accessible educational information for consumers

Health-Serving Organizations

The best way to locate a trusted source is to start at *www.healthfinder.gov*. Or check out the Medical Library Association, Consumer and Patient Health Information Section—top 100 Web sites you can trust (*http://caphis.mlanet.org/consumer/index.html*). Here are a few of the non-profit groups online and is by no means a complete listing:

American Academy of Family Practitioners (*www.familydoctor.org*)
American Cancer Society (*www.cancer.org*)
American Diabetes Association (*www.diabetes.org*)
American Dietetic Association (*www.eatright.org*)
American Heart Association (*www.americanheart.org*)

American Lung Association (*www.lungusa.org*)

Medem—content from a network of medical societies including the American Medical Association and American Academy of Pediatrics (*www.medem.com*)

National Mental Health Association (*www.nmha.org*)

The Nemours Foundation, Kids Health (*www.kidshealth.org*)

NOAH: New York Online Access to Health (*www.noah-health.org*)

Tufts Center on Nutrition Communication, Nutrition Navigator (*www.navigator.tufts.edu*)

University of California, San Francisco, HIV InSite (*http://hivinsite.ucsf.edu*)

Books

Albom, Mitch. *Tuesdays with Morrie: An Old Man, a Young Man, and Life's Greatest Lesson.* Doubleday, 1997. The hero of this book is Dr. Morrie Schwartz, a beloved professor dying of Lou Gehrig's disease. The story is motivational, inspirational, and provides guidance to patients and families dealing with tough issues.

Armstrong, Lance. *It's Not About the Bike: My Journey Back to Life.* Berkley, 2001. Lance Armstrong's story is well known to all of us. He was near death with far-advanced cancer of the testicle, which had spread into his brain, his lungs and his upper body. With aggressive surgery and chemotherapy, Lance has been cancer-free for many years. His feat is remarkable in and of itself, but he also is a four-time winner of the Tour de France, the most demanding endurance contest in the world of cycling. This story has courage, fortitude, perseverance and resiliency in the face of all odds.

Becker, Marty, D.V.M., with Danelle Morton. *The Healing Power of Pets: Harnessing the Amazing Ability of Pets to Make and Keep People Happy and Healthy.* Hyperion, 2002. We animal people know the truth about cats and dogs. My friend Dr. Becker clearly spells out the incredible bond between animals and us.

Kemper, Donald W., and Molly Mettler. *Information Therapy: Prescribed Information as a Reimbursable Medical Service.* Healthwise, 2002. The premise is to provide the right information to the right person at the right time. Shows how the Internet can deliver health information through doctors, health plans and hospitals. Companion Web site: *www.informationtherapy.org*.

Wolinsky, Howard, and Judi Wolinsky. *Healthcare Online for Dummies: Find the Facts and Advice You Need—Fast.* Hungry Minds, 2001. Already outdated Web sites but useful for research techniques in finding Dr. Right, the best hospitals, and navigating health insurance.

Exercise

Fenton, Mark. *Walking Magazine's Complete Guide to Walking for Health, Weight Loss, and Fitness.* Lyons Press, 2001.

Jordan, Peg. *The Fitness Instinct: The Revolutionary New Approach to Healthy Exercise That Is Fun, Natural, and No Sweat.* Rodale Press, 1999.

Kimiecik, Jay. *The Intrinsic Exerciser: Discovering the Joy of Exercise.* Houghton Mifflin, 2002.

Nelson, Miriam. *Strong Women Stay Young.* Bantam Doubleday, 2000. (Also look for *Strong Women Stay Slim* and others by Dr. Nelson in this series.)

Sweetgall, Robert. *Pedometer Walking: A New Look at Walking, Longevity, Weight Management, and Active Living.* Creative Walking, 2001 (*www.creativewalking.com*).

Nutrition

Rolls, Barbara, and Robert A. Barnett. *Volumetrics: Feel Full on Fewer Calories.* Harper Collins, 2000.

Stress

Adams, Patch, and Robin Williams. *House Calls: How We Can All Heal the World One Visit at a Time.* Reed, 1998.

Benson, Herbert. *The Relaxation Response.* Avon, 1990.

Benson, Herbert, and William Proctor. *Beyond the Relaxation Response: How to Harness the Healing Power of Your Personal Beliefs.* Berkley, 1994.

Eliot, Robert S., M.D. *From Stress to Strength: How to Lighten Your Load and Save Your Life*. Bantam, 1994. (Two classics if you can find them—see next book.)

Eliot, Robert S., M.D., and Dennis L. Breo. *Is It Worth Dying For? A Self-Assessment Program to Make Stress Work for You, Not Against You*. Bantam Doubleday, 1991.

Frankl, Viktor. *Man's Search for Meaning*. Washington Square, 1997.

———. *Man's Search for Ultimate Meaning*. Perseus Press, 2000.

Kabat-Zinn, Jon. *Wherever You Go, There You Are: Mindfulness Meditation in Everyday Life*. Hyperion, 1995.

Pachter, Barbara, with Susan Magee. *The Power of Positive Confrontation: The Skills You Need to Know to Handle Conflicts at Work, Home, and in Life*. Marlowe & Company, 2000.

Disease Management

Hagen, Philip, M.D. (editor). *Mayo Clinic Guide to Self-Care: Answers for Everyday Health Problems*. Kensington, 1999. (A family guide for every home on the basics.)

Wiebers, David, M.D. *Stroke-Free for Life: The Complete Guide to Stroke Prevention and Treatment*. Cliff Street Books, 2001.

Creagan, Edward T., M.D. (editor). *Mayo Clinic on Healthy Aging: Answers to Help You Make the Most of the Rest of Your Life*. Kensington, 2001. (I edited this book in a timely series from Mayo Clinic on various conditions such as depression, high blood pressure, managing diabetes, prostate health and more.)

Behavior Change

Prochaska, James O., John C. Norcross, and Carlos Diclemente. *Changing for Good*. Avon Books, 1995.

Seligman, Martin. *Learned Optimism: How to Change Your Mind and Your Life*. Pocket Books, 1998.

Seligman, Martin. *Authentic Happiness: Using the New Positive Psychology to Realize Your Potential for Lasting Fulfillment*. Free Press, 2002.

Cancer Specifically

Good for You! Reducing Your Risk of Developing Cancer (foreword by Edward T. Creagan, M.D.). American Cancer Society, 2002.

Eyre, Harmon, Dianne Lange, and Lois B. Morris (editors). *Informed Decisions: The Complete Book of Cancer Diagnosis, Treatment, and Recovery.* American Cancer Society, 2001.

Spiegel, David. *Living Beyond Limits.* Random House, 1995.

Contact the Author

Please understand that I cannot diagnose or review your personal medical information, but I welcome your feedback and comments through the Web site for this book at *www.HowNotToBeMyPatient.com*.

CHAPTER NOTES

Chapter 1: The Race Against Time

AARP (2002). *Beyond 50: A Report to the Nation on Trends in Health Security,* May 21.

Blendon, R. J. and colleagues (2001). "Americans' health priorities: Curing cancer and controlling costs." *Health Affairs* (Millwood). Nov-Dec; 20(6): 222–32.

Creagan, E. T. (2002). "The disease Americans fear most, why they don't have to." Health-eheadlines Consumer Health News Service (*www.health-eheadlines.com*).

Moynihan, R., I. Heath, and D. Henry (2002). "Selling sickness: The pharmaceutical industry and disease mongering." *British Medical Journal,* Apr 13; 324(7342): 886–91.

Oeppen, J., and J. W. Vaupel (2002). "Demography. Broken limits to life expectancy." *Science,* May 10; 296(5570):1029–31.

Scott, Joy (2002). "The impact of the baby boomers on healthcare marketing." *HealthLeaders.com,* May 8.

Society for Women's Health Research, Fact Sheet (*www.womens-health.org*).

Chapter 2: Pack Your Own Parachute

Barzilai, D. A., and colleagues (2001). "Does health habit counseling affect patient satisfaction?" *American Journal of Preventive Medicine,* Oct 24; 33: 595–99.

Dubbert, P. M. (2002). "Physical activity and exercise: Recent advances and current challenges." *Journal of Consulting and Clinical Psychology,* 70 (3): 526–36.

Dunn, A. L., and colleagues (2002). "Comparison of lifestyle and structured interventions to increase physical activity and cardiorespiratory fitness: A randomized trial." *The Journal of the American Medical Association,* Jan 27; 281(4):327–34.

McClure, J. (2002). "Are biomarkers useful treatment aids for promoting health behavior change? An empirical review." *American Journal of Preventive Medicine,* Apr; 22(3):200–7.

Prochaska, James O., John C. Norcross, and Carlos Diclemente (1995). *Changing for Good.* New York: Avon Books.

Chapter 3: Exercise: The Real Fountain of Youth

Andersen, R. E., and colleagues (1998). "Can inexpensive signs encourage the use of stairs? Results from a community intervention." *Annals of Internal Medicine,* Sept 1:129(5): 363–9.

Institute of Medicine, National Academy of Sciences (2002). "Dietary Reference Intakes for Energy, Carbohydrate, Fiber, Fat, Fatty Acids, Cholesterol, Protein, and Amino Acids (Macronutrients)." September (*www.iom.edu*).

Jordan, P. (1999). *The Fitness Instinct: The Revolutionary New Approach to Healthy Exercise That Is Fun, Natural, and No Sweat.* Rodale Press.

Malek, M. H., and colleagues (2002). "Importance of health science education for personal fitness trainers." *Journal of Strength and Conditioning Research,* Feb; 16(1):19–24.

Manson, J. E., and colleagues (2002). "Walking compared with vigorous exercise for the prevention of cardiovascular events in women." *New England Journal of Medicine,* Sept 5; 347(10):716–25.

Nelson, M. E., and colleagues (1994). "Effects of high-intensity strength training on multiple risk factors for osteoporotic fractures. A randomized controlled trial." *The Journal of the American Medical Association,* Dec 28; 272(24): 1909–14.

Perini, R. and colleagues (2002). "Aerobic training and cardiovascular responses at rest and during exercise in older men and women." *Medicine & Science in Sports & Exercise,* Apr; 34(4): 700–8.

Sands, W. A., and J. R. McNeal (2002). "A kinematic comparison of four abdominal training devices and a traditional abdominal crunch." *Journal of Strength and Conditioning Research,* Feb; 16(1):135–41.

Surgeon General (1996). Report on Physical Activity and Health: A Report of the Surgeon General.

Wei, M., and colleagues (1999). "Relationship between low cardiorespiratory fitness and mortality in normal-weight, overweight, and obese men." *The Journal of the American Medical Association,* Oct 27; 282(16):1547–53.

Chapter 4: Nutrition: You Are What You Put in Your Grocery Cart

Fuchs, C. S., and colleagues (2002). "The influence of folate and multivitamin use on the familial risk of colon cancer in women." *Cancer Epidemiology, Biomarkers and Prevention,* Mar; 11(3): 227–34.

Harris, G. K., and colleagues (2001). "Effects of lyophilized black raspberries on azoxymethane-induced colon cancer and 8-hydroxy-2'-deoxyguanosine levels in the Fischer 344 rat." *Nutrition and Cancer;* 40(2):125–33.

Kral, T. V., and colleagues (2002). "Does nutrition information about the energy density of meals affect food intake in normal-weight women?" *Appetite,* Oct; 39(2):137–45.

Rolls, B. J., (2000). "The role of energy density in the overconsumption of fat." *Journal of Nutrition,* Feb; 130 (2S Suppl): 268S–271S.

Rolls, B. J., and colleagues (2002). "Portion size of food affects energy intake in normal-weight and overweight men and women." *The American Journal of Clinical Nutrition,* Dec; 76(6): 1207–13.

Rolls, B. J. and L. S. Roe (2002). "Effect of the volume of liquid food infused intragastrically on satiety in women." *Physiology & Behavior,* Aug; 76(4-5): 623–31.

Sacks F. M., and colleagues (2001). "Effects on blood pressure of reduced dietary sodium and the Dietary Approaches to Stop Hypertension (DASH) diet. DASH-Sodium Collaborative Research Group." *The New England Journal of Medicine,* Jan 4; 344(1):3–10.

Sbrocco, T., and colleagues (1999). "Behavioral choice treatment promotes continuing weight loss: Preliminary results of a cognitive-behavioral decision-based treatment for obesity." *Journal of Consulting and Clinical Psychology,* Apr; 67 (2): 260–6.

Tordoff, M. G., (2002). "Obesity by choice: The powerful influence of nutrient availability on nutrient intake." *American Journal of Physiology,* May; 282(5):R 1536–9.

Wang, G., and colleagues (2002). "Economic burden of cardiovascular disease associated with excess body weight in U.S. adults." *American Journal of Preventive Medicine,* Jul; 23(1):1–6.

Xing, N., and colleagues (2001). "Quercetin inhibits the expression and function of the androgen receptor in LNCaP prostate cancer cells." *Carcinogenesis,* Mar; 22(3): 409–14.

Chapter 5: Deal with Reasonable Chaos and Gain Strength Through Stress

Amick, B. C., III, and colleagues (2002). "Relationship between all-cause mortality and cumulative working life course psychosocial and physical exposures in the United States labor market from 1968 to 1992." *Psychosomatic Medicine,* May-Jun; 64(3): 370–81.

Berk, L. S., and colleagues (1989). "Neuroendocrine and stress hormone changes during mirthful laughter." *American Journal of the Medical Sciences,* Dec; 298(6):390–6

Berk, L. S., and colleagues (2001). "Modulation of neuroimmune parameters during the eustress of humor-associated mirthful laughter." *Alternative Therapies in Health and Medicine,* Mar; 7(2): 62–76.

Eliot, Robert S., (1994). *From Stress to Strength: How to Lighten Your Load and Save Your Life.* New York: Bantam.

Eliot, Robert S., and Dennis L. Breo (1991). *Is It Worth Dying For? A Self-Assessment Program to Make Stress Work for You, Not Against You.* New York: Bantam Doubleday.

Grandey, A. A. (2000). "Emotion regulation in the workplace: A new way to conceptualize emotional labor." *Journal of Occupational Health Psychology,* Jan; 5(1): 95–110.

Karasek, R., and colleagues (1998). "The Job Content Questionnaire (JCQ): An instrument for internationally comparative assessments of psychosocial job characteristics." *Journal of Occupational Health Psychology,* Oct; 3(4):322–55.

Maruta, Toshihiko, and colleagues (2002). "Optimism-pessimism assessed in the 1960s and self-reported health status 30 years later." *Mayo Clinic Proceedings,* Aug; 77(8): 748–53.

Surwit, R. S., and colleagues (2002). "Hostility, race, and glucose metabolism in nondiabetic individuals." *Diabetes Care,* May; 25(5): 835–9.

Chapter 6: Lifestyle: Choice Not Chance

American Academy of Allergy, Asthma and Immunology and the Environmental Protection Agency. Smoke Free Home Pledge Campaign (*www.aaaai.org*).

American Cancer Society. Facts about secondhand smoke and restaurants (*www.cancer.org*).

Baker, F., and colleagues (2000). "Health risks associated with cigar smoking." *The Journal of the American Medical Association,* Aug 9; 284 (18): 2320–1.

Barendragt, J. J., and colleagues (1997). "The health care costs of smoking." *The New England Journal of Medicine,* Oct 9; 337(15):1052–7.

Brady, M. S., and colleagues (2000). "Patterns of detection in patients with cutaneous melanoma." *Cancer,* Jul 15; 89(2):342–7.

Breslow, L., and N. Breslow (1993). "Health practices and disability: Some evidence from Alameda County." *American Journal of Preventive Medicine,* Jan; 22(1): 86–95.

Cigarette Smoking among Adults—United States, 1999. *MMWR* 2001 Oct 12; 50 (40):869–73.

Creagan, E. T. (1997). "Malignant melanoma: An emerging and preventable medical catastrophe." *Mayo Clinic Proceedings,* Jun; 72(6):570–4.

Dale, L. C., and colleagues (2002). "Bupropion for the treatment of nicotine dependence in spit tobacco users: A pilot study." *Nicotine and Tobacco Research,* Aug; 4(3): 267–74.

Gansky, S. A., and colleagues (2002). "Oral screening and brief spit tobacco cessation counseling: A review and findings." *Journal of Dental Education,* Sep; 66(9): 1088–98.

Haddock, C. K., and colleagues (1999). "An examination of cigarette brand switching to reduce health risks." *Annals of Behavioral Medicine,* Spring; 21(2):128–34.

Kaplan, M.S. and colleagues (2002). *Journal of Gerontology: Medical Sciences* Jun; 57(6):M343–6.

Kramer, A., and colleagues (2001). "Regulation of daily locomotor activity and sleep by hypothalamic EGF receptor signaling." *Science,* Dec 21; 294 (5551):2511–5.

Martin, G. C., and colleagues. *Journal of the American Dental Association* 1999 Jul; 130 (7):945–54.

Mikkilineni, R., and colleagues (2001). "Impact of the basic skin cancer triage curriculum on providers' skin cancer control practices." *Journal of General Internal Medicine,* May; 16:302–7.

Muhn, C. Y., and colleagues (2000). "Detection of artificial changes in mole size by skin self-examination." *Journal of the American Academy of Dermatology;* 52 (5, pt 1):754–9.

National Highway Traffic Safety Administration. Drowsy Driving and Automobile Crashes (*www.nhlbi.nih.gov/health/prof/sleep/drsy_drv.pdf*).

National Institute on Aging. Exercise: A Guide from the National Institute of Aging, 1999 (*www.nih.gov/nia*).

Nunnez, N. P., and colleagues. "Alcohol consumption promotes body weight loss in melanoma-bearing mice." *Alcoholism: Clinical & Experimental Research,* May; 26(5): 617–26.

Oliveria, S. A., and colleagues (2001). "Skin cancer screening and prevention in the primary care setting: National Ambulatory Medical Care Survey 1997." *Journal of General Internal Medicine;* 16:297–301.

Perkins, K. A. (2001). Smoking cessation in women. Special considerations. *CNS Drugs;* 15(5): 391–411.

Rohrbaugh, M. J., and colleagues (2001). "Couple dynamics of change-resistant smoking: Toward a family consultation model." *Family Process,* Spring; 40(1):15–31.

Saraiya, M., and colleagues (2002). "Sunburn prevalence among adults in the United States, 1999." *American Journal of Preventive Medicine,* Aug; 23(2):91–7.

Shiffman, S., and colleagues (2000). "Efficacy of the nicotine patch for relief of craving and withdrawal 7-10 weeks after cessation." *Nicotine Tobacco Research,* Nov; 2(4):313–5.

Spangler, J. G., and colleagues (2002). "Tobacco intervention training: Current efforts and gaps in U.S. medical schools." *The Journal of the American Medical Association.* Sep 4; 288 (9):1102–9.

Taylor, S., and B. Diffey (2000). "Simple dosage guide for suncreams will help users." *British Medical Journal,* Jan 15; 320(7228):176–7.

Tomar, S. (2002). "Snuff use and smoking in U.S. men. Implications for harm reduction." *American Journal of Preventive Medicine.* Oct; 23(3):143.

Vachon, C. M., and colleagues (2001). "Investigation of an interaction of alcohol intake and family history on breast cancer risk in the Minnesota Breast Cancer Family Study." *Cancer,* Jul 15; 92 (2):240–8.

Winickoff, J. P., and colleagues (2003). "A smoking cessation intervention for parents of children who are hospitalized for respiratory illness: The Stop Tobacco Outreach Program." *Pediatrics,* Jan; 111(1):140–145.

Zhang, Z. F., and colleagues. (1999). "Marijuana use and increased risk of squamous cell carcinoma of the head and neck." *Cancer Epidemiology, Biomarkers & Prevention.* Dec; 8(12):1071–8.

Zhu, S. H., and colleagues. (2002). "Evidence of real-world effectiveness of a telephone quitline for smokers." *The New England Journal of Medicine,* Oct 3; 347(14):1087–93.

Chapter 7: What Should I Get Screened For—How and When?

Barry, M. J. (2001). "Prostate-specific-antigen testing for early diagnosis of prostate cancer." *The New England Journal of Medicine,* May 3; 344 (18):1373–7.

Chapple, A., and colleagues (2002). "Why men with prostate cancer want wider access to prostate specific antigen testing: Qualitative study." *British Medical Journal,* Oct 5; 325(7367): 725–6.

Discovery Health Channel–American Cancer Society Cancer Poll, 1999.

Etzioni, R., and colleagues (2002). "Overdiagnosis due to prostate-specific antigen screening: Lessons from U.S. prostate cancer incidence trends." *Journal of the National Cancer Institute,* Jul 3; 94(13):981–90.

Harris, R., and K. N. Lohr (2002). "Screening for prostate cancer: An update of the evidence for the U.S. Preventive Services Task Force." *Annals of Internal Medicine,* Dec 3; 137(11):917–29.

Laine C. (2002). "The annual physical examination: Needless ritual or necessary routine?" *Annals of Internal Medicine,* May 7; 136(9):701–3.

Landers, Susan J. "Full-body scans: Buying peace of mind." *amednews.com,* Sept. 3, 2001.

Morris, C. R., and colleagues (2001). "The risk of developing breast cancer within the next 5, 10, or 20 years of a woman's life." *American Journal of Preventive Medicine,* Apr; 20(3):214–8.

Oboler, S. K., and colleagues (2002). "Public expectations and attitudes for annual physical examinations and testing." *Annals of Internal Medicine,* May 7; 136(9):652–9.

Recommended Adult Immunization Schedule—United States, 2002–2003. MMWR 2002 Oct 11; 51(40):904–8.

Stone, E. G., and colleagues (2002). "Interventions that increase use of adult immunization and cancer screening services: A meta-analysis." *Annals of Internal Medicine;* 136:641–51.

Susan G. Komen Breast Cancer Foundation national study of young women's health needs. Press release, Sept. 25, 2002.

Thomas, D. B., and colleagues (2002). "Randomized trial of breast self-examination in Shanghai: Final results." *Journal of the National Cancer Institute,* Oct 2; 94(19): 1445–57.

Zapka, J. G., and colleagues (2002). "Healthcare system factors and colorectal cancer screening." *American Journal of Preventive Medicine,* Jul; 23 (1):28–35.

Chapter 8: How to Talk So Your Doctor Will Listen

Anderson, Eric. "Physicians should go back to basics with their patients." *amednews.com,* Oct. 7, 2002.

Beck, R. S., and colleagues (2002). "Physician-patient communication in the primary care office: a systematic review." *Journal of the American Board of Family Practice,* Jan-Feb; 15(1):25–38.

Bell, R. A. and colleagues (2001). "Unsaid but not forgotten: Patients' unvoiced desires in office visits." *Archives of Internal Medicine,* Sep 10; 161(16):1977–84.

Blumenthal, David. (2002). "Doctors in a wired world: can professionalism survive connectivity?" *Milbank Quarterly,* 80(3):525–46, iv.

Blumenthal, D., and colleagues (1999). "The duration of ambulatory visits to physicians." *Journal of Family Practice,* Apr; 48(4):264–71.

Branch, W. T., and colleagues (2001). "The patient-physician relationship. Teaching the human dimensions of care in clinical settings." *Journal of the American Medical Association,* Sep 5; 286(9): 1067–74.

Chakravarthy, M. V., and colleagues (2002). "An obligation for primary care physicians to prescribe physical activity to sedentary patients to reduce the risk of chronic health conditions." *Mayo Clinic Proceedings* Feb; 77(2): 165–73.

Cockburn, J., and S. Pit (1997). "Prescribing behaviour in clinical practice: Patients' expectations and doctors' perceptions of patients' expectations—a questionnaire study." *British Medical Journal,* Aug 30; 315 (7107): 520–3.

Commonwealth Fund. Accessing Physician Information on the Internet. January 2002. Access it: *www.cmwf.org.*

Coulter, A., and colleagues (1999). Sharing decisions with patients: Is the information good enough? *British Medical Journal,* Jan 30; 318 (7179): 318–22.

Deveugele, M., and colleagues (2002). "Consultation length in general practice: Cross sectional study in six European countries." *British Medical Journal,* Aug 31; 325(7362):472.

Deyo, R. A. (2001). "A key medical decision maker: The patient." *British Medical Journal,* Sep 1; 323(7311):466–7.

Eaton, C., and colleagues (2002). "Direct observation of nutrition counseling in community family practice." *American Journal of Preventive Medicine,* Oct; 23(3):174.

Epstein, R. H. "Major medical mystery: Why people avoid doctors." *The New York Times,* Oct. 31, 2000.

Epstein, R. M., and E. M. Hundert (2002). "Defining and assessing professional competence." *The Journal of the American Medical Association,* Jan 9; 287(2):226–35.

Eysenbach, G., and colleagues (2002). "Empirical studies assessing the quality of health information for consumers on the World Wide Web: A systematic review." *The Journal of the American Medical Association,* May 22-29; 287(20):2691–700.

Eysenbach, G., and C. Kohler (2002). "How do consumers search for and appraise health information on the World Wide Web? Qualitative study using focus groups, usability tests, and in-depth interviews." *British Medical Journal,* Mar 9; 324(7337):573–7.

Eysenbach, G., and C. Kohler (2002). "Does the Internet harm health? Database of adverse events related to the Internet has been set up." *British Medical Journal,* Jan 26; 324(7331):239.

Fallowfield, L., and colleagues (2002). "Efficacy of a Cancer Research UK communication skills training model for oncologists: A randomised controlled trial." *Lancet,* Feb 23; 359(9307):650–6.

Ferguson, Tom (2000). "Online patient-helpers and physicians working together: A new partnership for high quality health care." *British Medical Journal,* Nov 4; 321(7269):1129–32.

Hilton, M. E., and colleagues (2001). "Improving alcoholism treatment across the spectrum of services." *Alcoholism, Clinical and Experimental Research,* Jan; 25(1):128–35.

Kanzler, M. H., and D. C. Gorsulowsky (2002). "Patients' attitudes regarding physical characteristics of medical care providers in dermatologic practices." *Archives of Dermatology,* Apr; 138(4):463–6.

Keating, N. L., and colleagues (2002). "How are patients' specific ambulatory care experiences related to trust, satisfaction, and considering changing physicians?" *Journal of General Internal Medicine,* Jan; 17(1):29–39.

Langewitz, W., and colleagues (2002). "Spontaneous talking time at start of consultation in outpatient clinic: Cohort study." *British Medical Journal* Sep 28; 325(7366):682–3.

Little, P., and colleagues (2001). "Preferences of patients for patient centered approach to consultation in primary care: Observational study." *British Medical Journal,* Feb 24; 322(7284):468–72.

March of Dimes. "Folic Acid and the Prevention of Birth Defects: A National Survey of Pre-Pregnancy Awareness and Behavior Among Women of Childbearing Age," 1995–2001.

Mechanic, D., and colleagues (2001). "Are patients' office visits with physicians getting shorter?" *The New England Journal of Medicine,* Jan 18; 344(3):198–204.

Pattenden, J., and colleagues (2002). "Decision making processes in people with symptoms of acute myocardial infarction: Qualitative study." *British Medical Journal,* Apr 27; 324(7344):1006–9.

Pew Internet & American Life. Vital Decisions: How Internet users decide what information to trust when they or their loved ones are sick (includes a guide from the Medical Library Association about smart health-search on the Internet). Access it: *www.pewinternet.org.*

Roter, D. L., and colleagues (2002). "Physician gender effects in medical communication: A meta-analytic review." *The Journal of the American Medical Association,* Aug 14; 288(6): 756–64.

Schommer, J. C., and colleagues (2002). "Interdisciplinary medication education in a church environment." *American Journal of Health-System Pharmacy,* Mar 1; 59(5):423–8.

Science Panel on Interactive Communication and Health of the Department of Health and Human Services. Wired for Health and Well-Being: The Emergence of Interactive Health Communication. April 1999. Access it: *www.health.gov/scipich/pubs/finalreport.htm.*

Stange, K. C., and colleagues (2002). "One minute for prevention: The power of leveraging to fulfill the promise of health behavior counseling." *American Journal of Preventive Medicine,* May; 22(4):320–3.

Stevens, Larry. "Patients are bringing you health information they found online. They won't let you just ignore that. So what do you do?" *American Medical News,* Oct. 11, 1999.

Whitlock, E. P., and colleagues (2002). "Evaluating primary care behavioral counseling interventions: An evidence-based approach." *American Journal of Preventive Medicine,* May; 22(4):267–84.

Williams, J. D., and P. S. Bhagat. "The role of gender in determining strength and nature of marketing relationships." Paper presented to the Society for Consumer Psychology, February 2001.

Wilson P. (2002) "How to find the good and avoid the bad or ugly: A short guide to tools for rating quality of health information on the Internet." *British Medical Journal,* Mar 9; 324(7337):598–602.

Chapter 9: What They Never Taught Me in Medical School

Adams, Damon. "Physicians are working more, enjoying it less." *amednews.com,* June 3, 2002.

Boodman, S. G. "No end to errors." *Washington Post,* Dec. 3, 2002.

Cooper, R. A., and colleagues (2002). "Economic and demographic trends signal an impending physician shortage." *Health Affairs* (Millwood), Jan-Feb; 21(1):140–54.

Cooper, R. A., and T. E. Getzen (2002). "The coming physician shortage." *Health Affairs* (Millwood), Mar-Apr; 21(2):296–9.

Creagan, E. T. (1993). "Stress among medical oncologists: The phenomenon of burnout and a call to action." *Mayo Clinic Proceedings,* Jun; 68(6):614–5.

Creagan, E. T. (1999). "Bombarded by stress. Healthy habits to avert burnout." *Minnesota Medicine,* Aug; 82(8):14–5, 49.

Inlander, Charles. "Warning: Your Hospital Can Make You Sick: How to Protect Yourself." *Bottom Line/Personal,* April 1, 2002.

Morrison, I (2000). "The future of physician's time." *Annals of Internal Medicine,* Jan 4; 132(1):80–4.

Pathman, D. E., and colleagues (2002). "Physician job satisfaction, dissatisfaction, and turnover." *Journal of Family Practice,* Jul; 51(7):593.

"Physician burnout: Packing your career survival kit" (interview with Edward T. Creagan, M.D.). *Mayo Alumni,* Fall/Winter, 1997.

Quinn, G. E., and colleagues (1999). "Myopia and ambient lighting at night." *Nature,* May 13; 399(6732):113–4.

Rennard, B. O., and colleagues (2000). "Chicken soup inhibits neutrophil chemotaxis in vitro." *Chest,* Oct; 118(4):1150–7.

Shanafelt, T. D., and colleagues (2002). "Burnout and self-reported patient care in an internal medicine residency program." *Annals of Internal Medicine,* Mar 5; 136(5):358–67.

Chapter 11: The Search for Health, Peace and Serenity in Complementary Medicine

Becker, Marty, and Danelle Morton. *The Healing Power of Pets.* New York: Hyperion, 2002.

Benson, Herbert. *The Relaxation Response.* New York: Avon, 1990.

Benson, Herbert, and William Proctor. *Beyond the Relaxation Response: How to Harness the Healing Power of Your Personal Beliefs.* New York: Berkley, 1994.

Bernardi, L., and colleagues (2001). "Effect of rosary prayer and yoga mantras on autonomic cardiovascular rhythms: Comparative study." *British Medical Journal,* Dec 22-29; 323(7327):1446–9.

Clair, A. A. (2002). "The effects of music therapy on engagement in family caregiver and care receiver couples with dementia." *American Journal of Alzheimer's Disease and Other Dementias,* Sep-Oct; 17(5):286–90.

Cousins, Norman. *Anatomy of an Illness as Perceived by the Patient: Reflections on Healing and Regeneration.* New York: Bantam Doubleday, 1991.

Eisenberg, D. M., and colleagues (1993). "Unconventional medicine in the United States. Prevalence, costs, and patterns of use." *The New England Journal of Medicine,* Jan 28; 328(4):246–52.

Eisenberg, D. M., and colleagues (1998). "Trends in alternative medicine use in the United States, 1990-1997: Results of a follow-up national survey." *The Journal of the American Medical Association.* Nov 11; 280(18):1569–75.

Eisenberg, D. M., and colleagues (2001). "Perceptions about complementary therapies relative to conventional therapies among adults who use both: results from a national survey." *Annals of Internal Medicine,* Sep 4; 135(5):344–51.

Kessler, R. C., and colleagues (2001). "The use of complementary and alternative therapies to treat anxiety and depression in the United States." *American Journal of Psychiatry,* Feb; 158(2):289–94.

Kessler, R. C., and colleagues (2001). "Long-term trends in the use of complementary and alternative medical therapies in the United States." *Annals of Internal Medicine,* Aug 21; 135(4):262–8.

Mayo Clinic. "Pets and your health: The power of puppy love." Access it: *www.mayoclinic.com.*

Moertel, C. G., and colleagues (1981). "A pharmacologic and toxicological study of amygdalin." *The Journal of the American Medical Association,* Feb 13; 245(6):591–4.

Moertel, C. G., and colleagues (1982). "A clinical trial of amygdalin (Laetrile) in the treatment of human cancer." *The New England Journal of Medicine,* Jan 28; 306(4):201–6.

Moertel, C. G., T. R. Fleming, E. T. Creagan, and colleagues (1985). "High-dose vitamin C versus placebo in the treatment of patients with advanced cancer who have had no prior chemotherapy. A randomized double-blind comparison." *The New England Journal of Medicine,* Jan 17; 312(3):137–41.

National Institutes of Health, National Center for Complementary and Alternative Medicine. "What is complementary and alternative medicine (CAM)?" Access it: *www.nccam.nih.gov.*

Patterson, R. E., and colleagues (2002). "Types of alternative medicine used by patients with breast, colon, or prostate cancer: predictors, motives, and costs." *Journal of Alternative and Complementary Medicine,* Aug; 8(4): 477–85.

Post, S. G., and colleagues (2000). "Physicians and patient spirituality: Professional boundaries, competency, and ethics." *Annals of Internal Medicine,* Apr 4; 132(7):578–83.

Puchalski, C. M., and colleagues (2000). "Physicians and patient spirituality." *Annals of Internal Medicine,* Nov 7; 133(9):748–749.

Reibel, D. K., and colleagues (2001). "Mindfulness-based stress reduction and health-related quality of life in a heterogeneous patient population." *General Hospital Psychiatry,* Jul-Aug; 23(4):183–92.

Weiger, W. A., and colleagues (2002). "Advising patients who seek complementary and alternative medical therapies for cancer." *Annals of Internal Medicine,* Dec 3; 137(11):889–903.

Chapter 12: Attitude Matters: The Psychology of Survival and Longevity

Allen, K., and colleagues (2002). "Cardiovascular reactivity and the presence of pets, friends, and spouses: The truth about cats and dogs." *Psychosomatic Medicine,* Sep-Oct; 64(5):727–39.

Bretscher, M. E., and E. T. Creagan (1997). "Understanding suffering: what palliative medicine teaches us." *Mayo Clinic Proceedings,* Aug; 72(8):785–7.

Cassileth, B. R., and colleagues (1991). "Survival and quality of life among patients receiving unproven as compared with conventional cancer therapy." *The New England Journal of Medicine,* Apr 25; 324(17):1180–5.

Creagan, E. T. (1994). "How to break bad news—and not devastate the patient." *Mayo Clinic Proceedings,* Oct; 69(10):1015–7.

Creagan, E. T. (1997). "Attitude and disposition: Do they make a difference in cancer survival?" *Mayo Clinic Proceedings,* Feb; 72(2):160–4.

Creagan, E. T. (1999). "Attitude and disposition: Do they make a difference in cancer survival?" *Journal of Prosthetic Dentistry,* Sep; 82(3):352–5.

Danner, D. D., and colleagues (2001). "Positive emotions in early life and longevity: findings from the nun study." *Journal of Personality and Social Psychology,* May; 80(5):804–13.

Krucoff, M. W., and colleagues (2001). "Integrative noetic therapies as adjuncts to percutaneous intervention during unstable coronary syndromes: Monitoring and Actualization of Noetic Training (MANTRA) feasibility pilot." *American Heart Journal,* Nov; 142(5):760–9.

Maruta, T., and colleagues (2002). "Optimism-pessimism assessed in the 1960s and self-reported health status 30 years later." *Mayo Clinic Proceedings,* Aug; 77(8):748–53.

Omah, D., and colleagues (2002). "Religious attendance and cause of death over 31 years." *International Journal of Psychiatry in Medicine,* 32(1):69–89.

Petticrew, M., and colleagues (2002). "Influence of psychological coping on survival and recurrence in people with cancer: systematic review." *British Medical Journal,* Nov 9; 325(7372):1066.

Strawbridge, W. J., and colleagues (1997). "Frequent attendance at religious services and mortality over 28 years." *American Journal of Public Health,* Jun; 87(6):957–61.

Strawbridge, W. J., and colleagues (2001). "Religious attendance increases survival by improving and maintaining good health behaviors, mental health, and social relationships." *Annals of Behavioral Medicine,* Winter; 23(1):68–74.

Vickers, A. J., and B. R. Cassileth (2001). "Unconventional therapies for cancer and cancer-related symptoms." *Lancet Oncology,* Apr; 2(4):226–32.

INDEX

ABOUT THE AUTHOR

Edward T. Creagan, M.D., is professor at the Mayo Clinic Medical School. He holds endowed chairs as the American Cancer Society Professor of Clinical Oncology and the John and Roma Rouse Professor of Humanism in Medicine. Most recently, he was named Outstanding Educator from the Mayo Clinic School of Continuing Medical Education and has received the Distinguished Mayo Clinician Award. He completed an elected term as president of the Mayo Staff.

Dr. Creagan received his medical training at New York Medical College and earned graduate degrees in internal medicine and oncology at the University of Michigan and the National Cancer Institute before joining the staff at the Mayo Clinic in Rochester, Minnesota, where he has endured over thirty Minnesota winters. He is board certified in internal medicine, medical oncology, and hospice medicine and palliative care.

He is the author of over four hundred scientific papers and has given an equal number of presentations throughout the world, including his home state of New Jersey. His columns on health, wellness and the mind–body connection have appeared in Midwestern newspapers.

Dr. Creagan is associate medical editor of *MayoClinic.com*, Mayo Clinic's online Web site for consumer health information. He is the editor of the book *Mayo Clinic on Healthy Aging*.

An avid marathoner and golfer, father of three sons, grandfather of one incredible little boy, Dr. Creagan and his wife, Peggy, and their dogs and cats live in Rochester, Minnesota.

Collaborator **Sandra Wendel** is an Omaha-based consumer health–information journalist. Literally a "screen" writer, her cyber health stories appear on the top health Web sites, including her own Health-eheadlines Consumer Health News Service (*www.health-eheadlines.com*). She is also senior project editor for *eMedicine.com* consumer health.

Health and Wellness

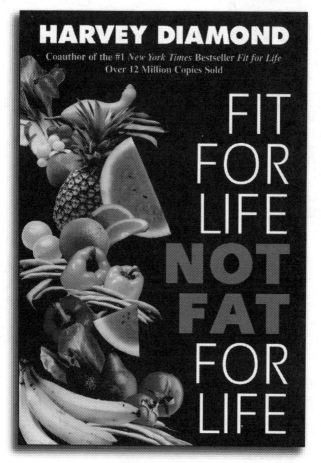

Code #1134 • Paperback • $14.95

Learn the secret to lifelong weight loss, wellness and longevity from the coauthor of the #1 *New York Times* best seller, *Fit for Life*. Includes new research, new ideas, new hope!

Body and Soul

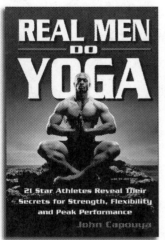

Code #1126 • Paperback • $12.95

Features 21 star athletes including NFL's Dan Marino, baseball's Barry Zito, the NBA's Kevin Garnett, plus pro golfers and tennis players.

Turn menopause into a positive and empowering experience, both physically and spiritually.

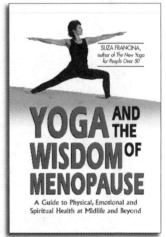

Code #0650 • Paperback • $12.95

Begin and maintain a yoga program with easy-to-follow instructional photos.

Code #4533 • Paperback • $11.95

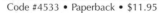